"The consequences of nurses mistreating and disrespecting each other are vividly recounted in this book. If nurses are to be caring and kind to patients, they must start with each other. Nurse managers can be critical to this effort. By learning to be part of the solution, rather than contributing to the problem, nurse managers can help both novices and experts maintain their commitment to civility and professionalism and a workplace free of tension and hostility."

–Suzanne Gordon, Author and Editor
First Do Less Harm: Confronting Inconvenient Problems in Patient Safety

When Chicken Soup Isn't Enough: Stories of Nurses Standing Up for Themselves, Their Patients, and Their Profession

"If only I had had this information when I was a manager, I wouldn't have had to lead by trial and error with bruised egos, wasted time, and energy-sucking melodrama to rival the best TV series. With its familiar vignettes and practical reflections, this book is a must-read for managers who understand that best practice means nothing if not embedded in a culture where every nurse feels emotionally secure. No human can think straight when upset. Managing toxic interactions is absolutely critical to patient safety. Toxic Nursing is worth every minute of your precious professional time."

–Kathleen Bartholomew, MN, RN
Nurse Leader, Consultant, and Author of
Ending Nurse-to-Nurse Hostility

"A wonderfully creative and comprehensive text designed to assist nurse managers in dealing with disruptive behaviors in the workplace. Scenarios are realistic, and commentaries are right on! Additionally, the self-reflective questions at the end of each scenario provide just-in-time strategies for nurse managers and provide invaluable insight as to how one's own or another's behaviors contribute to a healthy work environment (or lack thereof) and what to do about it."

–Lynda Olender, MA, NEA-BC, RN
Director of Nursing and Patient Care Services
Rockefeller University Hospital

"Toxic Nursing is a must-read for nurse managers, nurse preceptors, and new nurses. Dellasega and Volpe provide a comprehensive toolkit of approaches to address destructive workplace behaviors among nurses. The combination of vignettes based on cases gleaned from blog postings, and thorough literature review, is novel and effective. It will broaden the reader's view of 'bullying,' how it harms nurses and those they serve, and what to do about it."

–Anita J. Tarzian, PhD, RN
Associate Professor, University of Maryland School of Nursing
Program Coordinator, Maryland Health Care
Ethics Committee Network

Toxic Nursing

Managing Bullying, Bad Attitudes, and Total Turmoil

Cheryl Dellasega, PhD, RN, CRNP, and
Rebecca L. Volpe, PhD

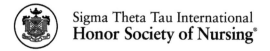

Sigma Theta Tau International
Honor Society of Nursing®

The Honor Society of Nursing, Sigma Theta Tau International (STTI) is a nonprofit organization whose mission is to support the learning, knowledge, and professional development of nurses committed to making a difference in health worldwide. Founded in 1922, STTI has 130,000 members in 86 countries. Members include practicing nurses, instructors, researchers, policymakers, entrepreneurs and others. STTI's 487 chapters are located at 663 institutions of higher education throughout Australia, Botswana, Brazil, Canada, Colombia, Ghana, Hong Kong, Japan, Kenya, Malawi, Mexico, the Netherlands, Pakistan, Portugal, Singapore, South Africa, South Korea, Swaziland, Sweden, Taiwan, Tanzania, United Kingdom, United States, and Wales. More information about STTI can be found online at www.nursingsociety.org.

Sigma Theta Tau International
550 West North Street
Indianapolis, IN, USA 46202

To order additional books, buy in bulk, or order for corporate use, contact Nursing Knowledge International at 888.NKI.4YOU (888.654.4968/US and Canada) or +1.317.634.8171 (outside US and Canada).

To request a review copy for course adoption, email solutions@nursingknowledge.org or call 888.NKI.4YOU (888.654.4968/US and Canada) or +1.317.634.8171 (outside US and Canada).

To request author information, or for speaker or other media requests, contact Rachael McLaughlin of the Honor Society of Nursing, Sigma Theta Tau International at 888.634.7575 (US and Canada) or +1.317.634.8171 (outside US and Canada).

ISBN: 9781937554422   EPUB ISBN: 9781937554439
PDF ISBN: 9781937554446   MOBI ISBN: 9781937554453
First Printing, 2013

Library of Congress Cataloging-in-Publication Data
Dellasega, Cheryl, author.
  Toxic nursing : managing bullying, bad attitudes, and total turmoil / Cheryl Dellasega and Rebecca L. Volpe.
     p. ; cm.
  Includes bibliographical references.
  ISBN 978-1-937554-42-2 (alk. paper) -- ISBN 978-1-937554-43-9 (EPUB) -- ISBN 978-1-937554-44-6 (PDF) -- ISBN 978-1-937554-45-3 (MOBI)
  I. Volpe, Rebecca L., 1983- author. II. Sigma Theta Tau International, issuing body. III. Title.
  [DNLM: 1. Nursing--organization & administration. 2. Personnel Management--methods. 3. Agonistic Behavior. 4. Bullying. 5. Interprofessional Relations. 6. Nurse's Role--psychology. WY 30]
  RT89.3
  362.17'3068--dc23
                              2013007411

Publisher: Renee Wilmeth
Acquisitions Editor: Emily Hatch
Editorial Coordinator: Paula Jeffers
Copy Editor: Kate Shoup
Proofreader: Barbara Bennett
Indexer: Jane Palmer

Principal Book Editor: Carla Hall
Development Editor: Emily Hatch
Project Editor: Brian Herrmann
Cover Designer: Alan Berry
Interior Designers: Rebecca Batchelor and
    Aleata Halbig

Dedication

To all the nurses out there who strive to make nursing the very best profession it can possibly be: We see you, too.

Acknowledgments

It takes a village to birth a book. Many wonderful minds contributed to this project, foremost among them our wonderful, thoughtful commentators—without them, there would be no book.

We also would like to thank Mary Lou Kanaskie and Justin Dennis for their feedback at the early stages of this project. They helped us keep our feet on the ground and our minds at the bedside.

To Kathy Curci for going the extra mile on more than one occasion, and to JSW for becoming an author.

Finally, last but by no means least, we must thank the men in our lives: Thank you for loving us, supporting us, and believing in us.

About the Authors

Cheryl Dellasega, PhD, RN, CRNP

Cheryl Dellasega is a professor in the Department of Humanities at the Penn State College of Medicine. She obtained her RN at Lancaster General Hospital, her BSN at Millersville State University, her MS and CRNP at the University of Delaware, and her PhD from Temple University. She is the award-winning author of the nonfiction books *Surviving Ophelia*, *Girl Wars*, *Mean Girls Grown Up*, *The Starving Family*, *Forced to Be Family*, and *When Nurses Hurt Nurses*. Her current clinical work is with adolescent girls through her programs Club and Camp Ophelia. Her research on geriatric nursing, psychosocial aspects of health, and relational aggression has been widely published and presented to international audiences.

Rebecca L. Volpe, PhD

Rebecca Volpe is an assistant professor in the Department of Humanities at the Penn State College of Medicine, as well as director of the Clinical Ethics Consultation Service for the Milton S. Hershey Medical Center. She earned her PhD from Saint Louis University's Center for Health Care Ethics and then went on to complete a Clinical Ethics Fellowship at California Pacific Medical Center. Her research interests include organizational ethics issues, such as organizational cynicism in hospital employees, and power/hierarchy in the medical setting. She is also interested in ethics education, including topics such as teaching students and providers moral methods, exploring effective evaluation strategies, and training currently practicing members of ethics committees.

Commentators

G. Rumay Alexander, EdD, RN
Clinical Professor and Director–Office of Multicultural Affairs
University of North Carolina at Chapel Hill School of Nursing

Lori S. Bechtel, MSN, RN
Nurse Manager, Neuroscience Critical Care Unit
Penn State Milton S. Hershey Medical Center

Peggy Ann Berry, MSN, RN, COHN-S, SPHR
PhD Candidate
University of Cincinnati

Beth Boynton, RN, MS
Organizational Development Consultant, Speaker, and Author
Beth Boynton, RN, MS Consulting Services

Theresa Brown, BSN, RN, OCN
Staff Nurse and Writer
Urban Teaching Hospital; *The New York Times*

Cheri Clancy, MSN, MS, RN, NE-BC
Director of Ambulatory Nursing, St. Christopher's Hospital
for Children
BSN Leadership Instructor, University of Medicine and Dentistry of New Jersey, School of Nursing

Katherine M. Curci, PhD, CRNP, CNM
Assistant Professor, Department of Family and Community
Medicine
Co-Medical Director, Penn State Hershey Medical Group at
Fishburn

Deana Deeter, CRNP, CHPPN, CPON
Hummingbird Program Manager
Penn State Milton S. Hershey Children's Hospital

Cheryl Dellasega, PhD, RN, CRNP
Professor of Humanities, Penn State College of Medicine
Professor of Women's Studies, Penn State University

Kelly K. Dineen, RN, JD
Assistant Dean for Academic Affairs
Instructor of Health Law
Saint Louis University School of Law

Cole Edmonson, DNP, RN, FACHE, NEA-BC
Vice President, Patient Care Services; Chief Nursing Officer
Texas Health Presbyterian Hospital Dallas
Robert Wood Johnson Foundation Executive Nurse Fellow

Patricia Artley Hart, MS, RN, CPN, NE-BC
Director of Nursing
Children's Hospital and Women's Health
Penn State Hershey Medical Center

Kathleen Merrill Jackson, DEL, MSN, RN
Doctoral Fellow and Consultant
Mountain State University and ITT Educational Services

Susan Johnson, MN, RN
Instructor; Doctoral Student
University of Washington

Mary Lou Kanaskie, MS, RN-BC, AOCN
PhD Candidate; Clinical Nurse Educator–Oncology
Nurse Residency Program Coordinator
Nursing Education and Professional Development
Penn State Milton S. Hershey Medical Center

Donna Kandsberger, MSN, RN, CPHON, PCNS-BC
Clinical Nurse Specialist, Pediatric Hematology/Oncology
Penn State Hershey Children's Hospital
Clinical Instructor, Department of Pediatrics
Penn State College of Medicine

Karlene Kerfoot, PhD, RN, NEA-BC, FAAN
Kerfoot & Associates, Inc.

Sherry Kwater, MSM, BSN, RN
Chief Nursing Officer
Penn State Milton S. Hershey Medical Center

Mary T. Meadows, MS, MBA, RN, CENP
Director, Professional Practice, AONE
Executive Director, AONE Foundation

Eric R. Messner, PhD, FNP-BC
Assistant Professor
Department of Family and Community Medicine
Penn State Milton S. Hershey Medical Center
Penn State College of Medicine

Victoria Schirm, PhD, RN
Director of Nursing Research
Penn State Milton S. Hershey Medical Center

Shellie Simons, PhD, RN
Associate Professor, Department of Nursing
University of Massachusetts Lowell

Melissa J. Snyder, DEd, CRNP
Campus Coordinator of Nursing Programs
Penn State Harrisburg

Isabelle St-Pierre, PhD
Assistant Professor, Department of Nursing
Université du Québec en Outaouais, Canada

Carol Tringali, MS, RN, AOCNS
Clinical Nurse Specialist, Hematology/Oncology
Penn State Milton S. Hershey Medical Center

Nancy Marie Valentine, PhD, MPH, RN, FAAN, FNAP
President, Valentine Group Health
Nurse Researcher, Lankenau Institute of Medical Research
Adjunct Associate Professor, University of Pennsylvania School
of Nursing

Dilek Yildirim, PhD, RN
Associate Professor, Gazi University, Health Science Faculty
Nursing Department
Besevler/Ankara/Turkey

Table of Contents

Introduction

We live in an era of complex care and adversarial administration. In times gone by, the "head nurse" was in charge of a unit; now the person in charge is expected to "manage." In the past, longevity often determined who was or was not promoted; now, senior staff may have more experience in the classroom than in the "real world" of work. A diverse workforce further complicates the job of the nurse leader on both micro and macro levels.

Conflict, which can be transient or ongoing, intense or mild, personal or professional, also challenges nurse leaders, particularly on the management level of administration. Although few managers receive education on conflict resolution, most confront it on a daily basis in one form or another.

Conflict exists on many levels and for many reasons. Tension may trickle down from the top or bubble up from below, and while it is individually defined, a nurse manager must have the capacity to handle conflicts that can create a toxic work environment. Johansen (2012) links the ability of nurse managers to address inter- and intrapersonal stress among coworkers with the quality of patient care.

To better offer an understanding of conflict management in the nursing workplace, we conducted a review of problems reported in the scholarly literature. Then, to explore nursing perspectives more intimately, narratives rather than research or anecdotal articles were selected for review. Specifically, blogs were used as a source of stories shared by nurses.

In early 2012, a Google search was run using the terms "nurse bullying" and "nurse conflict and cynicism." There were 6,300,000 hits for "bullying" and 10,200,000 for "conflict." A review of the top 100 sites for each category of the two searches revealed that blogs on bullying evoked many more responses, with only one blog specific to conflict and chaos.

To identify blogs that would provide content on common nursing conflicts, the following criteria were used. First, they had to be about nurses in practice, not students. Second, there needed to be more than three posts from different posters featured on the blog. Third, the blogs had to refer to nurses or situations related to the nursing profession within the United States. Finally, they had to be written in English. Using these guidelines, 21 useable blogs were identified.

The number of posts on the 21 blogs ranged from 3 to 431. All were signed anonymously, i.e., using a first name or screen name. Some of the posts were in response to a query about the topic of conflict and/or bullying, while others were written in response to a previous post or news story.

The selected blogs were further reviewed, with each post numbered consecutively. The authors then read each post individually and independently to analyze them for themes related to conflict, cynicism, or chaos.

Once all posts had been reviewed and assigned to a theme, we met to discuss the themes identified on each post. These were then collapsed and categorized into larger content areas of metathemes (categories), which became the 16 chapters of this book. Where there was disagreement, we discussed and, if consensus couldn't be reached, a third reviewer was asked to provide input.

A third independent nurse/reviewer was asked to read exemplar posts assigned to each theme and to agree or disagree with the assignment. This reviewer and another nurse/administrator/reviewer then reviewed the final categories to confirm that they captured "real life" sources of conflict at the workplace.

Narrative "vignettes" were then constructed based on each theme, with the exception of four vignettes, which were submitted to the authors specifically for inclusion in this book. Each vignette was compared to original blog posts emerging from the specific theme for veracity. Further, we compared vignettes with 50 written narratives shared during workshops, lectures, and email correspondence as a further confirmation of validity.

By coincidence, Gaffney, DeMarco, Hofmeyer, Vessey, and Budin (2012) published the results of their narrative analysis of stories about "bullying," which were received online from 99 nurses. The results of their study are one more confirmation of the validity of our themes in that stressful situations described were almost identical to the ones we identified through our blog review. That is, a thematic analysis of the stories submitted to Gaffney and her colleagues revealed that hazing/humiliation by a preceptor, intimidation, name calling, abuses of authority, use of patient assignments to mistreat, accusations of subpar performance, retaliation, exclusion, gossip, judging, ignoring, and/or threatening loss of their jobs were all sources of bullying for the nurses who volunteered to describe real-life situations.

For this book, after the vignettes were developed, 27 experts in nursing management were asked to comment on the narratives from the perspective of preventing, addressing, or minimizing the consequences of conflict. These experts were identified through personal contacts, literature review, and recommendations from colleagues. Experts were asked to avoid citing references and rely on their own expertise and intuitive skills to provide practical advice about the situation.

Each chapter, organized in relation to a theme identified through the blogs, provides a brief introduction, the vignettes, and at least two expert commentaries. Although the process used to generate vignettes was not rigorous or categorized as scientific research, it was conducted using a thoughtful and scholarly process that would lead to valid conclusions. The commentary of experts was lightly edited without altering the actual content to preserve the "real life" context.

Valentine (2005) found that nurse managers often relied on "compromise" to address conflict. This book suggests that a range of skills are required to fully address nursing conflicts and the adverse outcomes that can result. Communication, problem solving, support measures, reframing, education, and awareness raising, as well as assessment, consultation, and collaboration, were all behaviors identified by experts as key across different areas of conflict.

Although intended for nurse managers specifically, it is our hope that nurses in other positions will find the content in this book useful. Continued personal and professional growth and improvement lead to a goal valued by all nurses: the best possible patient care.

— Cheryl Dellasega and Rebecca L. Volpe

part I bitter behavior

1 | the newbie: mistreatment of new nurses

"Mature nurses" are the new "new nurses." The traditional career trajectory for nurses used to be graduation from high school and immediate entry into a diploma or college program for nursing. After graduation, the new nurse would most likely head off to a hospital job that would last for many years, if not all of his or her work life. Such a homogenous group led to a different type of integration into the workplace.

Now, there are multiple educational paths and a diverse assortment of nurses entering the nursing profession. According to the Bureau of Labor Statistics, the most common route into nursing is as an associate-degree nurse, with 26% more nursing jobs predicted for the future (2012). Jobs for nurses will continue to be plentiful and increase at a faster rate than other professions. At the same time, nurses may not be as happy as in the past.

A large survey of nurses found that nearly half planned to leave their job within the next 3 years. Kearns (2010) also notes that "almost 50% of the respondents were nurses between the ages of 40–49, and 59% of the nurses currently hold a position on their hospital's permanent staff." Further, 8% of nurses were returning to the workforce, many for economic reasons. These trends all lead to a much more fluid workplace, varied motivations for seeking employment, greater complexity in coordinating care, and the need for nurse managers to be extremely flexible and versatile.

Consider a typical orientation program at a community hospital. Among the new employees are:

- Sara, a 38-year-old medic, who served in Iraq and returned to school for her BSN. She will be working part-time in the ED while continuing to take classes to become a nurse practitioner.

- Luke, a 27-year-old veterinary assistant who worked his way through a 2-year AD program. His dream is to be an OR nurse, but he has followed the advice of a friend to "get some experience" and taken a position on the same-day surgery unit.

- Marci and Bette, both aged 22 and freshly graduated from a 4-year program and thrilled at the prospect of their first job. They have accepted positions on a busy surgical floor.

- Annette, a 40-year-old mom, is reentering the workplace after her husband lost his job. A diploma nurse, she has worked part-time as a school nurse but now is headed full-time for a medical unit.

One can easily imagine how challenging it will be to meet the orientation needs of this diverse group, especially with the demand to cover so many required policies and procedures. Meeting the needs of "nontraditional" nurses can be a critical determinant of retention since the "fail to complete" orientees are often dissatisfied with the climate of their new workplace (Dellasega, Gabbay, Durdock, & Martinez-King, 2009).

Among the conflicts a nurse manager confronts, none can be as disheartening as the "eating our young" phenomenon (Dellasega, 2009). The literature, the Internet, and the hospital cafeteria are rife with stories about new nurses being hazed, harassed, and treated as "odd nurse out" (Gaffney, DeMarco, Hofmeyer et al., 2012). In their analysis of 81 narratives, these authors found that "being the newbie" was often associated with bullying.

However, a study of 511 randomly selected new RNs by Simons (2008) found no statistical difference in bullying between seasoned and new nurses. For either group, bullying was a significant predictor of intent to leave, and therefore actual turnover. The problems most often reported were unmanageable workload, being ignored or excluded, and having opinions disregarded.

We found that nurses identified conflicts such as RNs with a diploma (i.e., 3-year) education believing they should be "grandfathered" in and considered the same as nurses with an associate or baccalaureate degree. Not only was this suggestion insulting to the new nurse with a hard-earned university degree, it caused a divide between nurses from different educational backgrounds.

Another challenge was that incoming orientees had skills and abilities from their previous jobs that might be relevant to various aspects of nursing practice—budgeting or communication skills, for example. However, their knowledge wasn't respected because they were "new to nursing." This not only deflated the self-esteem of the second-career nurse, but it was a potential waste of valuable resources.

The nurse preceptor was frequently discussed in relation to new graduates. Younge, Hagler, Cox, and Drefs (2008) discovered in their mailed survey to more than 80 nurse preceptors that this role was challenging and often unappreciated. Hrobsky and Kersbergen (2002) found the same: Nurses who acted as preceptors for new graduates found the experience stressful, especially when the encounter was not successful. They received no extra pay or recognition for an assignment that added to their already substantial workload.

Many of the comments we read described negative situations for preceptees. Sometimes, older nurses precepted younger nurses in a way that seemed more critical than helpful, with a kind of "popularity contest" occurring. Those nurses who were not "liked" found themselves being targeted by others and even set up to fail.

Commentator Cheri Clancy notes,

> *If conflicts are not resolved properly or if there is not a "zero tolerance" policy in place for poor behavior, many new nurses may observe and embrace the bullying behaviors of other nurses just to fit in. Sadly, this creates an acculturation, or the continuation of bullying behavior.*

Vignettes, Commentaries, and Reflective Thinking

The remainder of this chapter presents vignettes about new nurses experiencing mistreatment, commentaries about the experiences represented in the vignettes, and opportunities to explore or reflect on the material.

Vignette 1.1: Just As Good

Rosemary is right out of college and proud of the BSN she earned through hard work, perseverance, and encouragement from her parents, who took out several loans to finance her education. Her first job is on a postsurgical floor at General Hospital, where most of her coworkers are older and long-term employees at the institution.

Rosemary is the newest nurse on the unit. During orientation, her preceptor, Eilene, comments frequently on the differences between a nurse with an associate degree and one with a BSN.

"Why go to school for so long?" she asks Rosemary in front of a group of nurses. "I have an AD and I've done just fine. They ought to just grandfather us in."

"That's right," another nurse with the same background adds. "Forget all this encouragement to get a 4-year degree. We know just as much as they do."

Rosemary begins to feel targeted by comments from Eilene and other coworkers. She questions whether she really did make the right choice in obtaining a 4-year degree and becomes anxious about her performance.

Expert Commentary: Vignette 1.1

I would start by having a conversation with Rosemary to explain why some of the older nurses are feeling this way. They aren't really targeting her personally, but it's a reflection of a lack of understanding on their part.

To a degree, there is some validity to what Eilene and the other nurses are saying. Initially, there is a basic understanding common to BSN and AD nurses. What Rosemary needs to keep in the back of her mind is that over time, her ability to think and see beyond the basic technical functions will become evident.

It may also be a lack of exposure to nurses with advanced degrees that makes the other nurses feel as if there is no difference. Rosemary needs to value the experience of her new co-workers but also remember that she brings a piece to this work environment that they do not have. The nurse manager needs to tell them the new nurse might have something to teach them, too.

The other thing the nurse manager needs to do is have a conversation with all of the older nurses (including the preceptor) and let them know that while they are valued for their experience, they need to remember this is a new nurse, and they were new nurses at one time, too. They need to guide and support her in the way they wanted to be guided and supported.

A general rule is don't judge a person by the initials at the end of the name.

–Kathy Curci

The topic of ADN versus BSN nurses is a "great debate" among many. Unfortunately, the mere mention of this topic to two or more nurses will likely end in a heated discussion. Arguably, there are many pros and cons of various entry-level options in the nursing profession. Despite some program differences, both ADN and BSN graduates sit for the NCLEX-RN exam and are held to the same rigid standards for licensure and practice. The caveat to this vignette is that seasoned ADN nurses, such as Eilene and her colleagues, may feel threatened by this push for higher education in nursing because many organizations now hire or promote only BSN-prepared RNs. Obtaining a BSN is admirable and offers many pros such as job security, research-/evidence-based practice concepts, and an overall broad knowledge base. As many health care organizations are in a quest for Magnet designation, one mandate is the percentage of nurses who must hold a BSN in that organization. The BSN also provides students with an introduction to research and how to apply evidence-based practice to nursing care. Having extensive courses in psychology or other humanities also brings the BSN-prepared nurse an eclectic knowledge base, which will help strengthen critical-thinking skills. This is not to say the ADN does not have these attributes. The ADN may indeed have acquired this through self-learned practice and continuing education. However, in the era of "proving oneself," the lack of such a degree unfortunately supersedes ones credibility.

Rosemary, the new BSN, is now faced with trying to defend her degree while preserving her preceptor's dignity and credentials. The last thing Rosemary wants to do is damage her relationship with her colleagues or appear to be better positioned in the organization due to her higher degree. It may benefit Rosemary to acknowledge both the pros and cons of her degree to avoid undermining or overrating herself. Sharing her feelings and concerns with her mentors may be the best remedy to an awkward situation. For example, Rosemary could state that while she is proud of her degree and looks forward to sharing her knowledge to help move the unit forward, she is really eager to learn and grow from practical experiences set forth by Eilene and her other colleagues. New BSN graduates need to position themselves as confident in their educational pathways, yet very curious in the quest to learn from those senior to them, regardless of degree. Working toward a "team approach" rather than a "me approach" is the key to overcoming degree dichotomies. Both seasoned and unseasoned RNs have opportunities to learn from one another.

—Cheri Clancy

Reflection

How do you handle a mix of educational backgrounds on your unit? When there's tension between different subgroups of nurses, are you inadvertently drawn into supporting the ones who are most like you, or most like your own background?

Do you believe there is a difference between nurses with 2, 3, or 4 years of education? How do you, as a leader, adjust your style to address these differences, if at all?

Vignette 1.2: The *Right* Kind of Experience

Coretta is eager to succeed at her first job in the operating room (OR)—a position she has dreamed of since she first entered nursing school. She has gone through orientation and is now working as a "real" nurse after passing her boards.

As a student, Coretta did a review of the literature on handwashing procedures used in the OR for one of her classes and got an A from her professor. During her first month on the job, she makes some subtle suggestions to her coworkers, based on what she learned from the research for her paper.

"Are you kidding?" responds Helen, who has worked as an OR nurse for 25 years. "Is that what they teach you in college? Wait until you have some experience under your belt, and then you can give other people advice."

From that point on, Coretta is labeled a "know-nothing" nurse. Every time she questions why a procedure is done a certain way, her coworkers roll their eyes. At her first evaluation, her nurse manager suggests that Coretta should focus on learning from her more experienced coworkers.

Coretta emails one of her professors and tells her about the situation: "I feel like all my classes count for nothing! Maybe nursing isn't the right profession for me."

Expert Commentary: Vignette 1.2

I think that the nurse manager really needs to step in here. This is a learning opportunity for Coretta. Coretta may need to time things differently and wait until she is there longer. She could be guided to build a relationship and earn respect before she suggests that they could do things better.

It's not clear why Coretta would expect things to be any different. She needs to respect the fact that the unit has its own ways of doing things that have been in place for a long time. They may even have ways that are more effective. Just because something is in the literature doesn't necessarily mean that it's practical and works with real patients or for a particular unit. I tell my students, "Your patient didn't read the literature."

I would probably take a step back and say something to the older nurses to prevent a divide, too. Coretta is making suggestions in an effort to help, not to suggest she knows more than the other nurses. Her motives are genuine. All of us in our enthusiasm have probably done this very thing. Everyone goes into a new job with great ideas.

–Kathy Curci

Behaviors such as hostility and undermining are considered forms of bullying. To effectively deal with bullying in the workplace, it is important to set aside emotions and place emphasis on the facts. The most important person who can stop this bullying is Coretta. Coretta should keep a record of the times when Helen or other colleagues make an inappropriate comment or exhibit an inappropriate behavior. It is important to document the time, place, person, and actual occurrence, being cognizant to only write the facts. Eye rolling, fist slamming, or other inappropriate nonverbal behavior should also be documented.

Some bullies feel threatened or are intimidated themselves, so Coretta should assess her own comfort level before approaching the bully (or bullies). One major mistake some nurses make when confronted by a bully is to try to reason with the bully and attempt to convince the bully he or she is wrong. It is important not to be nice, but rather remain professional and firm when speaking to the bully. Being nice may confirm to the bully that he or she is in a superior position.

If Coretta chooses to approach Helen or the other bullies, she should state the facts in a mutually agreed-upon place. Sometimes, when bullies are presented with data rather than drama (crying, yelling, etc.), they may actually recognize the inappropriateness of their behavior—especially if there is documentation and quotes. If Coretta feels her dialogue with Helen didn't go well, or if she is uncomfortable speaking directly with Helen, Coretta should report her findings to her nurse manager and even the human resources department. Informing management (in writing) and documenting all occurrences and any previous attempt to resolve the issue at the lowest level is vital.

The term "hostile work environment" is a legal term in the workplace. When formally documenting, use words such as "bullying," "hostile work environment," and "intimidation." Coretta should continue to seek support from others to release some of her stress as a result of the bullying.

–Cheri Clancy

Reflection

When an employee is excited to implement a new project, at what point do you feel a nurse manager might be led to intervene, and how? What guidelines help you differentiate between needed change and the hubris of an inexperienced employee?

What things do you put in place to create a culture of continual learning? As a nurse manager, do you value evidence-based practice, and, if so, how do you help your employees to realistically use these principles in everyday practice?

Vignette 1.3: Not So New

Lisa graduated from college with a degree in biology and went to work in a lab. After a few years, she realized that she didn't really enjoy what she was doing, so she decided to quit her job and go back to school for a nursing degree. Lisa completed an 18-month BSN program, and, at age 31, started her first nursing job.

The problems began at the very beginning—during orientation. She was in a group of new-grad orientees, which meant that everyone was almost a decade younger than she was. Other new grads looked at her askance and didn't seem to want to talk to her.

The worst part was that Lisa felt like she was treated like a complete know-nothing. While venting to her husband one night, she said, "I mean, I realize I'm new to nursing, and that most of my colleagues spent more than 18 months on their nursing degrees, but it feels like my whole prior career just didn't matter at all!"

It's not that Lisa feels like she's better than her new-grad colleagues. It's just that she has a whole host of skills as a result of being in the workforce for a decade (interpersonal relations, professionalism, people skills, etc.), and she is really upset that she's treated like a know-nothing in every respect.

Expert Commentary: Vignette 1.3

The other nurses in the orientation group don't know Lisa and don't understand what her previous degree is all about. How would they know?

Truthfully, she needs to take a step back and say, "I may have a degree and work experience elsewhere, but it's unrealistic to think that others would understand that." Most of the other nurses being oriented may not have a lot of experience themselves, and their contact with patients might have been as student nurses. They're not at a point in terms of professional maturity to appreciate the added skills Lisa may bring.

They don't know how that will play out in patient interactions; no one really does.

–Kathy Curci

Nursing as a second career is becoming very popular. Second-career nurses are entering the profession with diverse work experience and educational backgrounds, and this diversity strengthens the nursing profession. These nurses are adult learners who bring a variety of talents to the nursing profession with their different life and work perspectives. More-seasoned nurses should be cognizant that although they may be senior to these new nurses, they also have an opportunity to learn from these new nurses' previous skills. Employment skills such as critical thinking, emotional intelligence, customer service, and computer skills easily transfer to the nursing profession.

It is important that Lisa shares her experiences with her colleagues. New-nurse orientation can be very intimidating and filled with mixed emotions by many attendees. Lisa can begin gaining respect from her colleagues and even adopt a mentor role by sharing her prior experiences in the lab and applying this to the clinical setting.

–Cheri Clancy

Reflection

As nurses on your unit accomplish goals such as continued education or increased skill level, how do you respond? Is it appropriate for the nurse manager to acknowledge achievements and endorse particular steps his or her employees take to improve their performance?

How do you feel about nurses who take online courses or work toward a higher degree be given different responsibilities because they are trying to advance their careers? Is the seasoned, "tried and true" employee the one you turn to when rewards are being handed out or the one who seeks continuing education?

Vignette 1.4: Popularity

The 23-hour unit has a high turnover with a diverse group of nurses who seem to come and go quickly. Lauren, an RN who has been on the unit since it was created, is the designated preceptor for new employees.

Beth, Lauren's latest charge, is right out of school and has a habit of laughing when she's nervous. Halfway through their second day together, Lauren is extremely frustrated and tells her coworkers that Beth isn't taking her feedback and suggestions seriously. Her comments get more pointed.

"Get with it, girl," Lauren tells Beth, who accidentally enters information in the wrong place. "This is the world of high tech. You should be better at computers than me!"

Later that week, Beth allows a patient to choose between two pain medication options the physician ordered. Lauren overhears the conversation and takes Beth aside as soon as she leaves the patient's room. "Never let a patient choose for himself! They don't know anything about these medications—you're the nurse!"

When Beth laughs and says she's sorry, Lauren sighs and walks away. Later, at lunch, she tells her coworkers that she thinks Beth is a "problem" because she isn't taking the job seriously.

Expert Commentary: Vignette 1.4

I would hope that Lauren, the preceptor, could develop a better understanding of how people handle stress and be able to identify that Beth wasn't really laughing, but was simply attempting to cope. Maybe the conversation needed to occur right up front. Lauren might say, "I notice when you get nervous you laugh. Is that really what's happening?" This will validate what she's seeing. From that point forward, others would know that Beth's laughter is not making fun of them, nor does it indicate Beth is not taking them seriously.

I would say that if this progresses and Lauren says things like, "Never let a patient choose for themselves," Beth needs to ask, "Why was that a wrong decision?" Otherwise the comment won't have credibility. Then Lauren needs to sit down with Beth and give her feedback on her rationale. She could tell Beth that the nurse knows the pharmacology and can make a better choice than the patient. The physician doesn't give choices to the patient; the physician gives them to the nurse so he or she can make the best decision. That's part of developing your clinical practice: making important decisions and judgments.

Given the way this situation unfolded, Beth, really learned nothing from the feedback. It's the preceptor's job to help the new nurse grow and develop.

–Kathy Curci

Emotional intelligence (EI) is not an innate attribute, but a learned skill that must be nurtured and developed. EI is the ability to identify your own emotions, use your emotions constructively, understand emotions in uncomfortable or hostile situations, and manage one's own emotions and those of others to achieve positive outcomes. Nurses' emotions play a vital role in nurse-patient perceptions as well as mentor-preceptor interactions. Because Lauren is in a preceptor role, it is vital that she be in sync with Beth's comfort level. Beth's nervous laughter could have been handled more effectively had Lauren had EI training. With proper leadership training and EI competence, Lauren could have identified the situations or antecedents that triggered Lauren's laughter and provided more time in teaching, explaining, or demonstrating the skill.

Leaders that lack leadership competence and emotional competence cannot effectively manage others. Although nurses possess emotional intelligence in varying degrees, if it is fragmented, it can create an unhealthy workplace environment. In a healthy workplace environment, leaders are attuned to their emotions and the emotions of others in various situations. Incorporating EI training as part of the preceptor or leadership training programs is paramount for successful nurse leadership.

–Cheri Clancy

Reflection

Behavioral tics, mannerisms, or other responses to stressful situations can be traumatic for those who have them and misunderstood by colleagues who only see the outward behavior. What is your responsibility as a nurse manager when such behaviors occur?

At what point are personal behaviors unacceptable? For example, if you have an employee whose loud voice, overbearing presence, or other habits create discord among your staff, how do you intervene, knowing that productivity is being disrupted?

Vignette 1.5: Trial By Fire

Dr. Smith is a surgeon known for his short temper and curt comments to nurses. While the nurses on the postsurgical unit are used to this mistreatment, they fail to tell Anne, a new nurse, that Dr. Smith expects a prompt report on his patients when he walks into the room, including the latest set of vital signs.

One day, Dr. Smith enters a room where Anne is working. When Anne continues what she is doing and doesn't acknowledge Dr. Smith, he pushes the bedside table away roughly, so he can examine the patient. "You need to go back to school and learn how to take care of patients who just had major operations!" he tells her. Then he addresses the patient: "These new nurses. It takes years before they're any good."

Wendy, one of Anne's more experienced coworkers, happens to walk by the room just then and laughs. "Dr. Smith is at it again," she tells the unit secretary.

Anne comes out of the room, clearly upset. She sees Wendy and asks what she did wrong. "Oh, you'll learn. Dr. Smith has his own way of doing things. We all went through one of his meltdowns," Wendy replies with a shrug of her shoulders.

Expert Commentary: Vignette 1.5

These kinds of incidents can sometimes be perceived as "paying your dues." It's been said that this is what you have to go through to get into this exclusive sorority. The same kind of hazing can happen if a nurse has special credentials or higher education.

Right away, the chief of staff needs to have a talk with Dr. Smith. The fact that nurses have patterned their behavior to allow his behavior to continue is really a disservice to everyone. He obviously has no respect for nurses, and his judgment of being "a good nurse" may be skewed. The fact that they snap to attention when he comes on the floor is not how I would judge a good nurse.

As the nurse manager, I would pull the nurses aside who let this poor person walk into a loaded situation and tell them I'm disappointed by their lack of support. Anne is part of this team, and the expectation is that they will work together and share information. Obviously, the nurse manager has supported this kind of behavior for it to go on and has allowed the nurses on her unit to act this way. The nurse manager needs to step up and tell Anne what's really going on.

Ultimately, the actions of nurses on a particular unit are a reflection of the nurse manager. She is responsible for the behavior of her staff.

–Kathy Curci

Creating a healthy workplace environment where nurses can speak up will increase staff morale and patient safety. Addressing inappropriate behavior when it occurs, if applicable, is the key to obtaining a healthy work environment. If Anne is thinking she is "just a staff nurse" and those acting inappropriately hold more power because of their position, then she should think again. This is a case where one person, Anne, the informal leader, can definitely make a difference. Staff nurses need to be patient advocates as well as team advocates. To accomplish this, Anne can address her concerns with Dr. Smith and her manager as soon as possible and in a private setting (not in front of patients), perhaps beginning by addressing her newness to the profession, as well as to the culture of the organization and the surgeon's preferences.

The National Labor Relations Act and the Occupational Safety and Health Administration (OSHA) give individuals the right to report incidents without losing their jobs or suffering other reprisals. Ensuring and maintaining a healthy work environment are responsibilities of all members of an organization. According to a recent Gallup poll, nursing has been the most respected profession for the past 7 years. This could not have been accomplished without earning the respect and trust of our patients and others.

All nurses need to fully support the American Nurses Association (ANA) Code of Ethics. The code of ethics states professional nurses have an ethical mandate to become skilled communicators. In order to embrace this mandate, every nurse needs to look within himself or herself first and make initial efforts to foster healthy workplace environments. Having effective nurse-physician collaborations among nurses, physicians, and health care leaders is critical to sustaining strong interdisciplinary and intradisciplinary relationships. The Joint Commission recommends adopting a zero-tolerance policy for intimidating and/or disruptive behaviors and to incorporate this into organizational policies, other medical bylaws, and employment agreements.

–Cheri Clancy

Reflection

Can your staff count on your prompt intervention to halt denigrating and disrespectful behavior from physicians or other personnel who use condescending and rude behaviors toward them?

Are nurse managers in your institution unified in their commitment to demanding a level of respect from other coworkers for yourselves and your employees? What actions have each of you taken to insure that nurses are given the same privileges and opportunities as physicians?

Summary

In addition to all the cultural and religious backgrounds that exist in one unit, educational backgrounds continue to be a major element of diversity within the nursing profession. Each individual brings his or her own experiences and knowledge to the unit regardless of education; however, in nursing, years of school is a delicate topic that some might argue fosters confusion, frustration, and bullying among new nurses and their seasoned colleagues.

Nurse managers can work with their staff to promote an environment of learning, communication, collaboration, and compromise. One nurse, while more experienced and perhaps more knowledgeable, is not automatically superior to her peers. By working together and respecting all ages and educational backgrounds, nurse managers can create a healthy working environment and offer better-quality care to their patients. The nurse manager's challenge is to (1) see the advantage of having a workforce of educationally diverse nurses on his/her staff, and then (2) promote a safe, diverse working environment.

One way to begin this task is to start with the preceptors. Select preceptors who are caring, informed, and proficient nurses—and overall great teachers. They must have respect for the new generations coming in as well as the knowledge and experience these "newbies" can bring to the unit. They must also know how to prepare new nurses for both the positive and negative realities of the profession and nurture their continued education for a better future.

Another idea is to work closely with your new nurses during their first several months of employment. Provide them with the tools they need to be successful in their career. Be their support system—make them feel comfortable discussing issues such as bullying with you. Show that you will provide them with some sort of resolution if they do share challenges such as relational aggression.

If we can address the source of the bullying problem, new-nurse retention should greatly increase. In order to change the culture of aggression that may have taken root on your unit, lead the way to change. Be an advocate for your staff, and provide an atmosphere of learning and appreciation. Help dismiss prejudices that exist with different educational backgrounds, and show your staff that each individual's strengths are what makes your unit operate on a daily basis.

Activities

If coworkers see each other as people as well as nurses, they are more likely to work collaboratively. Have each nurse write on a small index card one "fun fact" about his/her hobbies, interests, or talents, along with his/her name. Create a Bingo-type sheet with the reported fun facts in separate squares and ask new employees to find out who they belong to. When they meet the person who matches the fun fact, they can write down his or her name and X out the square containing it. When they have a line of names, they can come to you and receive a small prize or check off part of their orientation list.

Alternatively, have one of your mature staff members interview newbies for some basic fun information. The interviewer can then "introduce" the newbie at the next group meeting. Sample interview questions include "What do you like to do for fun?," "What made you go into nursing as a career?," and "How do you like to spend your birthday?"

2 | the know-it-all/ criticism queen

We may not think of nit-picking, fault-finding, and criticism as forms of bullying, but when they happen chronically, they certainly are. According to the Workplace Bullying Institute, workplace bullying is "repeated, health-harming, mistreatment of one or more persons (the targets) by one or more perpetrators." In addition, the Workplace Bullying Institute ("The WBI Definition of Workplace Bullying," 2012) states that this mistreatment can take one or more of the following forms:

- Verbal abuse

- Offensive conduct/behaviors (including nonverbal), which are threatening, humiliating or intimidating

- Work interference—sabotage—which prevents work from getting done

Scholars sometimes add to this definition the criteria that there must be a power differential, and that most victims of bullying struggle to defend themselves against bullies in large part because they find themselves lower on the workplace hierarchy than the bully (Dehue, Bolman, Vollink, & Mouwelse, 2012).

In their recent study on bullying in the workplace, Francine Dehue and her colleagues asked 361 people living in the Netherlands, "How often have you been unnecessarily criticized [at work]?" The results indicate that this is a not-uncommon problem. According to Dehue, 22% of respondents said they were unnecessarily criticized at work at least once a month. As though being unnecessarily criticized at work were not enough to try to deal with, people who said they were unnecessarily criticized on a frequent basis were more likely to have health complaints and to report depression (Dehue, et al., 2012).

There's an archetype of women in the workplace: the Queen Bee. This is the boss lady (think Miranda Priestly in *The Devil Wears Prada*) who claws her way to the top and does everything she can to undermine, put down, and generally squish other women who are trying to achieve the same level of success. Interestingly, recent research by Catalyst, a nonprofit organization that focuses on expanding opportunities for women in the workplace, seems to indicate that most women *don't* actually look at their female subordinates as competition that needs to be cut down or eliminated. Instead, they look at their junior female colleagues as potential talent—and, it turns out, are more likely than men to develop that talent through informal or formal mentorship (Catalyst, 2012; Gray, 2012).

And yet, somehow this study doesn't seem to ring true for nurses. We still seem to have "Supernurses," and these Supernurses still seem to have ego trips at the expense of our more junior colleagues. (Of course, not all Supernurses are women; plenty of men fit this mold, too.) The Catalyst study wasn't specifically looking at nurses, or even medicine. Perhaps this is one lesson that we can learn from our nonnursing colleagues: We should cherish, mentor, and cultivate our junior colleagues, not rip them to shreds. Unless we want to work until the day we die, we'll need someone to fill our roles when we retire!

Sometimes there may be a grain of truth in criticism, which has the unfortunate consequence of causing the target to believe that the entire criticism has validity. In turn, this can cause diminishing self-esteem and confidence of nurses at work. More often, though, instead of being based on a kernel of truth, the criticism is based on a distortion, fabrication, or misrepresentation. When this happens, victims have a choice: They can speak up or stay silent. If they speak up to defend themselves, they risk further mistreatment by the bully. If victims stay silent, this seems to implicitly sanction the bullying behavior, and it may slowly build resentment, frustration, and anger. It may also cause some social anxiety in victims, where they dread social situations and experience anxiety because they fear being unexpectedly criticized. This, in turn, can negatively affect job performance. After all, how can people be doing their best when they feel someone is constantly looking over their shoulder, trying to anticipate the next obscure, unnecessary criticism?

Commentator Peggy Ann Berry notes,

Bullying behavior, incivility, and disrespectful behaviors are endemic in the stressed environment of nursing. Leadership education on disruptive acts can help nursing staff understand the multiple root causes of bullying behavior and how to decrease the bullying behaviors through their own behavior or response.

Sometimes, however, leadership education alone is not enough. In some cases, the best approach is simply to have a frank conversation with the bully, and to tell that person about the emotional and economic consequences of his or her overly critical behavior. If bullies understand that there is a zero-tolerance policy for their behavior—and, the key, that the policy will actually be enforced—their behavior is much more likely to change.

There are no guarantees, though. Often, bullies have been bullies for much of their life, and changing lifelong habits can be difficult if not impossible. However, for the sake of our young nurses—our future leaders—we must do our very best to ensure that they are not chronically cowed by the know-it-all Supernurse.

Vignettes, Commentaries, and Reflective Thinking

The remainder of this chapter presents vignettes about bullying in the form of critcism, commentaries about the experiences represented in the vignettes, and opportunities to explore or reflect on the material.

Vignette 2.1: Extreme Criticism

Ron, the night nurse on the medical step-down unit, is fanatical about keeping patient rooms free of clutter. He identifies nurses who "leave a mess" at the change of shift and lectures them publicly.

After an especially busy evening shift, Deb, who juggled an extra patient due to short staffing, is preparing to go home—30 minutes late. Ron comes down the hall with a frown on his face. "Deb, I hope you're not leaving! Your patient in 670 has dirty linen all over his room!"

Rather than argue with Ron, Deb goes back to the room and discovers a used patient gown on the bathroom floor where the patient had left it after changing. She puts it in the laundry, but the next day she complains to the nurse manager about Ron's "pickiness" and public harassment.

Expert Commentary: Vignette 2.1

Observing the behavior of a single nurse within an organization is diagnostic of the style, needs, and wants of that individual, and how their personal and professional aspirations are being met (or not). It is also a window into an organization and how well it functions overall. The leadership expectations, the management accountabilities, and the social culture of the unit as well as of the organization on a larger scale are transmitted to employees, patients, and the community. All these elements reflect the values and expectations of the micro unit and macro organization, and are embedded in every behavior that staff display. That is why, in looking at the behavior of a single nurse, we must consider not only that individual but also the larger context in which that person is living, much like we would in considering the role of family dynamics in family therapy. There may be a "patient," but there is also the family that tolerates the individual and often, consciously or unconsciously, reinforces defiant or deviant behavior, therefore disrupting the entire family unit. Let's look at how these play out in practice.

Every employee has strengths and stresses from various areas of his or her life. Work can often be a stage for living out the drama of one's own life. In reading this example, I wonder if Ron has teenagers who are also leaving a mess at home? The difference between an unhealthy work environment and one that allows staff to work out conflicts in a healthy and productive way is that the unhealthy environment allows individuals to project blame, vent anger openly, and give license to an overall sense of lack of control. In essence there are no guidelines for conflict management that serve to solve problems and reinforce open, honest communication.

In this example, Ron appears to be the agent of control. On one hand, his desire to keep rooms free of clutter is a good thing, but is it a shared value for the team? When he roars, people tolerate the bad behavior but quickly lose sight of the fact that what he is trying to achieve may be worth considering. It is all in how the group decides to set expectations and share in the decision-making and accountability for making decisions reality.

What are the options here? Let's look at each role:

- **Deb:** Deb could talk to Ron directly, focusing on how Ron is inflating the problem—how she agrees with his objective, but not his method of communicating it. This could also offer the opportunity to have a broader discussion about room clutter at the next staff meeting. Deb does not react to the behavior, but can focus on the patient-centered objectives and how to create a more orderly environment for the benefit of all.

- **Ron:** Ron could identify room clutter as less of a personal objective than one that is focused on the patient from an aesthetic, quality, and infection-control perspective. He could take a leadership role with staff and explore with others the reality of how room clutter detracts from a professional environment that is aiming to provide patients and families with a four-star environment.

- **Unit manager:** The unit manager can listen to Deb without taking sides, instead seeing the situation as an opportunity to practice conflict-management techniques. He or she could use this example in a follow-up discussion with the entire team on how to resolve issues and set expectations that are fair, achievable, and attainable for all. By remaining nonreactive, the manager functions as a facilitator rather than an agent of control forcing the team to come to terms with each other. After a discussion on the issue of room clutter, staff-to-staff interactions, techniques to settle conflict, and how to respect each other, the manager in essence has moved the group to a different level of communication. The manager has also made expectations clear. Both have a role in making the unit a harmonious place to be. This serves as a baseline for future interactions between Ron and other staff.

If the behavior persists, Ron may need individual coaching to recognize his responsibilities to his teammates. A determination may need to be made as to whether he can remain on the team. At the same time, the group must take joint responsibility and not let its reactions go underground, thus reinforcing his negative approach. Ron must learn that his behavior is not acceptable, and everyone needs to understand the steps involved in how to handle such issues in the future. Ron will find he gets more cooperation from his peers when he approaches them as a peer rather than as a critical, harping superior. And team members will feel more in control, knowing that when conflicts arise, it is their responsibility to deal directly with each other and to work out problems together.

–Nancy M. Valentine

Nurse managers must deliberately practice good listening skills to all complaints pushed up to them by their employees. Pushing a problem up the chain of command isn't easily done by nurses. The culture has taught them to be silent or vent within their "safe" coworker groups. However, your main goal is to provide exceptional, safe patient care by empowered nurses. Keeping communication channels open will alert the nurse manager to problems brewing in the unit before a battle between shifts or units, or escalating nurse conflict, occurs. Open lines of communication are important.

Confronted with the report of Ron's behavior, the nurse manager knows any past attempts between peers has failed. Ron's peers have exhausted their tools to stop the behavior. Frustrated and angry about Ron's public cacophony, these nurses may avoid Ron at shift change. Peer communication has stopped, as well as any information required on change of shift.

Before acting, investigate! Speak to observers and targets of Ron's behavior. Begin a private discussion with Ron from his perspective and coach him on his behavior. A first-time complaint or observation may not require disciplinary action. A private conversation and coaching may uncover the basis of Ron's behavior and a gap on a professional communication standard between shift changes. Document your coaching interventions with Ron.

As a nurse manager, you should meet with each shift. Coaching and disciplinary action require your active involvement to change behavior. As a nurse manager, speak to all staff on your expectations at shift change. Create a policy and procedure with a checklist for shift change to ensure a consistent approach. And, as their manager, model the professional behavior you want to see in your staff. Unprofessional behavior disappears in the manager's presence, so be prepared to continue surveillance and keep communication open.

Formal disciplinary action is required if Ron's behavior persists. To continue coaching or disciplinary action, consult with human resources and employee health services. Human resources will counsel and strengthen your approach on coaching or progressive disciplinary action according to policy. Employee health services can schedule psychological counseling for the employee or unit, if needed.

–Peggy Ann Berry

Reflection

Do you think Ron's behavior counts as bullying? If not, why not? Identifying bullying can sometimes be difficult—and can feel like drawing an arbitrary line in the sand. Where do you draw that line in your unit? What do you do when a behavior might be right on the line, but not clearly over it?

As a nurse manager, what strategies can you use to work with Ron?

Vignette 2.2: Passing Judgment

The nurses on the labor and delivery (L&D) floor know that Tessa is openly critical of the emergency department (ED) and calls the nurses who work there "lazy and sloppy." One day, an emergency admission arrives on L&D just as Tessa is returning from lunch. As everyone hustles around the patient, Tessa grabs the chart and begins flipping through it.

"Just what I expected," she says to the patient's husband, who is standing near the room where his wife is being treated. "The ED nurses didn't get most of the information we need. Now I'll have to go through it all over again with you."

Tessa makes sure to tell the nurse manager what happened, along with complaining to the other L&D nurses about the ED's "crappy" patient care. The next time there is a transfer, the ED nurse makes sure to be as rude as possible to Tessa, and a unit-to-unit "feud" develops between the ED and L&D.

Expert Commentary: Vignette 2.2

Acting out feelings, even by one individual, rather than discussing problems openly is an indication of a team that is not functioning as a team—either on its own unit or between units. There are tension points in all jobs. Everyone has a responsibility to deal with conflicts in an adult manner, not display emotion as a child who throws a tantrum when she does not get her way.

In a family-centered care environment, the patient comes first, not a staff member's tension points. Judgmental behavior such as that displayed by Tessa communicates an "I don't want to work here with these incompetent people" attitude. This in turn communicates to the patient and her husband that they are being cared for by an organization that does not value excellence.

Otherwise, why would the hospital employ staff members who do not know what they are doing? Tessa's behavior puts everyone on the team and the organization as a whole at risk, as the patient and her husband potentially lose confidence at a time when they need their confidence to be reinforced. Respect for patients and a willingness to make them the center of all services must be an organizational value that is reinforced in all interactions. To deliver anything less is a violation of the trust that an employer places with the employee and the consumer expects from those in which care is entrusted.

What are the options?

Tessa is clearly angry and out of control. She is displaying unprofessional behavior to her coworkers and to the patient and the patient's husband. A staff member, manager, or supervisor needs to be brought into the discussion before the shift ends to review the outburst.

With the support of the unit manager, the L&D staff must confront Tessa about the issue with the ED staff. This can be done in a small group discussion and then followed up in a larger staff meeting. In conjunction with the managers of each of the units, "lazy and sloppy" work must be identified and remedied in a businesslike manner. A review of patient-centered care must be reinforced with all staff understanding how this is translated in practice. Language such as "crappy" patient care is not to be tolerated, and Tessa must receive an unequivocal warning that such behavior has to stop.

The unit, service, and organization as a whole must reinforce the values that are held. Policies, procedures, brochures, posters, and the strategic plan must reflect that patient- and family-centered care is the focus. This will serve to support staff members in their work. In addition, such value statements can be used in disciplining Tessa for her behavior, thus keeping her personally accountable and team members accountable to each other to uphold these values every day as they partner with each other and with those who are served.

–Nancy M. Valentine

Tessa has been openly critical at transfers (or handoffs) from ED to the L&D unit. These complaints are well known to her peers, and she has come to the nurse manager with the latest incident. Her continual complaints may or may not be justified. However, Tessa was unprofessional verbalizing her complaint in front of a laboring patient's husband.

First, it doesn't take much imagination to see a red-faced expectant father screaming at the ED staff after Tessa's statement. After a full investigation confirms a public complaint to the patient and husband, a written reprimand should be privately issued to Tessa. This written reprimand should also include instructions on immediate cessation of public criticism of the ED to her peers or anyone other than the manager. ED communication at transfer after the incident is obviously strained. As the nurse manager, you will be the one to bring the ED and the L&D staff together by apologizing for Tessa's behavior to the ED manager. This will begin to repair the breach to ensure professional communication is reinstated at transfer.

Second, does Tessa know how to constructively present complaints up the chain of command? Have her previous complaints been met with resistance to address issues? Do her complaints have merit on transfers from the ED to L&D? Handling Tessa's ongoing complaints constructively may reveal gaps in transfer. Ask her to bring solutions with her complaints. Determine if a transfer policy, procedure, or education is needed to meet the transfer needs of L&D and the ED. A new checklist that fairly addresses responsibilities between the ED and L&D on documentation and transfer to L&D may increase patient safety and decrease tension during handoff.

Successful channeling of staff complaints may create quality improvement with other processes. In my research, I have found that nurses who file complaints and see no change become increasingly disempowered or disgruntled by lack of action on management's part. Lack of trust in management related to poor follow-through on legitimate issues leads to silent resignation and disempowerment.

As a nurse manager, are you listening? When a problem or complaint comes up, how do you inform your staff of your actions to correct the problem? Do you consider the psychosocial and physical safety of your nurses a priority, given that nurse job satisfaction is correlated to patient satisfaction?

Are nurse managers the last to know? Yes, unless a nurse manager is on the floor on a continual basis interacting with his or her staff, conflicts and complaints can go unreported and unnoticed. This is because the culture has taught nurses to be silent to those in power. However, nurse managers need to promote expectations on open communication, encourage staff to bring solutions to address problems, and provide transparency with solving these complaints. The staff needs to know why issues can't be resolved yet or will never be resolved.

–Peggy Ann Berry

Reflection

It's so easy—in life and at work—to be critical of others. We sometimes think to ourselves: "If only *I* had been there, this could have been done right!" Yet there is so much we don't know about the reality of the situation, because we *weren't* there.

When nurses are critical of others, what can you do about it? What are some reasonable steps to take to try to help the criticism queen see that they might not have the complete story? If things progress further—into a feud—what strategies would you employ to try to mend fences with other units in your organization?

Vignette 2.3: Anything You Can Do, I Can Do Better

Although Maureen has worked in the MICU (medical intensive care unit) for only 2 years, the other nurses refer to her as "Supernurse." The nickname isn't meant as a compliment. "One time, I had just worked a double and had barely kept on top of my patients, who were both very unstable," recalls Sandy, a longtime MICU nurse. "When I was telling Maureen about it, she assured me that nothing could be worse than the time *she* worked a double and had two *even sicker* patients."

"Maureen actually did an online search and printed out information on this weird EKG pattern my patient had one day," says Terry, another MICU nurse. "She kept insisting she was right, even though it was a transient arrhythmia with no associated symptoms. During shift report, she made sure to mention her superior knowledge and made me look stupid."

Maureen's one-upmanship goes beyond her interactions with nurses. When physicians come into the MICU, she rushes to help them and makes sure they know how efficient and in control she is. None of her colleagues is quite as able or smart as she is—or so Maureen thinks.

Expert Commentary: Vignette 2.3

The idea of a "Supernurse" is a fantasy, as no one can "know it all" in today's fast-paced health care scene. Moving into an established work team can be very difficult even for experienced nurses, and it is just that much harder for a younger, inexperienced nurse to find a place on the team. One of the symptoms of an insecure and potentially anxious person is to call attention to one's own abilities and shut out others in the process. It is a self-fulfilling process of isolation and the antithesis of collaboration, which is essential in today's multidisciplinary approach to care. It may be that Maureen is overwhelmed by the level of illness of the patients in the MICU, and this is an unconscious mechanism that she is using to convince herself that she is in control and won't make an error in caring for such ill patients. Although it may come across as an ego trip, her insistence on being right may be a symptom of fear, not superiority.

To test out the hypothesis, a unit manager could connect with the senior nurses in a coordinated effort to informally reach out to Maureen, developing a closer relationship with her rather than being offended by her behavior (as annoying as it may be) and getting to know her beyond the specifics of her direct work with patients. It will take time, commitment, and a genuine interest in adopting Maureen to the team for this approach to work. The key to turning this around is for the nurse manager to remind the senior nurses not to take Maureen's comments personally but to be willing to dig deeper into what is causing her to act in this manner. Trying to get to know Maureen as an individual on a level of colleagueship rather than "upmanship" could help to lessen her anxiety and help her relax to the point where she can share in a more authentic manner. It is entirely possible that when she feels more comfortable, less on edge about how she has to "perform," she will openly share her concerns and be willing to learn from the experienced crew, who can teach her a lot of what she needs to know.

It is also important for the unit manager to review the orientation program for nurses new to a specialty unit. There is a great deal to absorb, and the support, coaching, and reinforcement of how the team works and how she can move comfortably into the team is a critical area of such an orientation.

The support role of the manager of the unit is critical to Maureen's success. Weekly meetings to explore how things are going, to formally review her behavior, and to coach her on alternatives could be very helpful to Maureen as well. She is clearly a babe in the woods on the way to Grandma's house. The senior nurses can either be the big, bad wolf and eat her up over time or take her under their collective wing and smartly show her the way to a satisfying career on the MICU. It is a choice; if the outreach is successful, the entire team will benefit and grow in the process.

In health care, working harmoniously with others' care is a challenge at every level, from staff nurse at the bedside to nurse executive in the boardroom. At every turn, there are difficult and demanding people whom you must "win over" to a healthier approach to communicating and engaging in the work at hand. Team development, positive reinforcement, and celebrating success go a long way to developing a culture where people are more willing to play together in the sandbox. It is a challenge and why nursing is a "practice" profession. We learn and grow every day.

–Nancy M. Valentine

That big "S" on Maureen's chest may stem from competition, insecurity, or even social exclusion by peers. Have coworkers constructively given her feedback on her behavior or silently witnessed it? They may have talked about Maureen's behavior among other nurses or have started to avoid talking or working with her. As the nurse manager, you may have seen her display the behavior or seen her peers scatter at her approach, which can and does affect patient and nurse safety.

Begin by documenting what you observed or heard her say. Start a private conversation with Maureen in your office to initiate coaching. Gently determine what the main issue is for her behavior. Coaching may be effective in eliminating Maureen's behavior, but it might not change coworkers' attitudes toward her. All staff must be educated on negative behaviors in the work environment and what professional behaviors are expected. As with Ron, if the behavior does not abate, begin additional disciplinary action.

We all need to be mindful of our behavior and reactions toward each other. Educate staff on appropriate responses to the perpetrator's behavior immediately, constructively, and assertively. If the power balance is apparent, the nurse manager must address the issue. Educate on assertive communication to stop the behavior before the cycle of disrespect, conflict, and bullying escalates. Speak to and post expected professional behavior and empower nurses to use the chain of command to help change the nursing culture.

–Peggy Ann Berry

Reflection

First, put yourself in Maureen's shoes. From a 10,000-foot perspective, how do you think she became the person she is today? Is it possible her behavior stems from insecurity? What can you, as the nurse manager, do to try to support the Supernurse so she doesn't feel the need to brag about how much better than everone else she is?

Next, think about the colleagues Maureen is chronically showing up. What can you do to support them? How must they feel? The nurse manager's challenge in this situation is to support these nurses without deepening the divide between colleagues.

Summary

Relational aggression (RA) uses words as weapons; this can mean being hypercritical, depreciating, or severe. RA can be linked with all kinds of adverse physical and psychological outcomes.

RA has sometimes been called "female bullying" because while males tend to aggress physically (or through war), women have a long history of using more covert, relational ways to express conflict.

It is the nurse manager's responsibility to create a climate of cooperation and respect on his/her unit. First, and perhaps most importantly, the nurse manager needs to role-model the kind of behavior(s) employees are expected to adopt. Next, each person must recognize that he or she has the potential to act out the behaviors of being too aggressive or too passive or standing by. Identifying specific situations that may provoke each type of behavior will help stimulate a discussion of helpful alternatives. As with most things, initiating a frank conversation on the unit about bullies, victims, and silent observers is a good place to begin.

There are, however, nurses who are always on the attack, stuck in what we call the "RA rut." No matter what the situation, this nurse is in aggressor mode—ready to humiliate, intimidate, or manipulate. The nurse manager should make use of careful documentation and confrontation when aggressive behaviors occur, so there is a record of either improvement or continued mistreatment of peers.

Finally—just remember that we are all *human*. We all have good days and bad; we all have deep, dark stories that cast light on why we are the way we are. We're *all* dysfunctional in some way. It's important to hold people accountable and take action to try to make things better. But, it's also important to remember that there is usually a relatively compelling story behind toxic behaviors.

Activity

The "Supernurse Syndrome" (Dellasega, 2009) occurs when one nurse believes he or she is automatically a better nurse and more skilled than everyone else. Are there Supernurses in your hospital? On your unit? By any chance, could you be a Supernurse?

Answer the following questions to explore further.

Using a scale of 1-10, with 10 "agree as much as possible" and 1 "disagree as much as possible," respond to the following:

- I believe that I am a very skilled nurse.
- My supervisors and other administrators consider me a good nurse.
- I am the best nurse in my organization.
- The feedback I get from my coworkers about my nursing abilities makes me feel as confident as possible.
- I am more skilled than most of my coworkers.

These questions are meant to prompt reflection on how you view your own competencies in comparison to those of your colleagues. You could also use them in a meeting of either colleagues or staff and start a dialogue on the Supernurse Syndrome.

3 | gossip and trash talk

In its 2001 report, *Crossing the Quality Chasm: A New Health System for the 21ˢᵗ Century,* the Institute of Medicine (IOM) committee on the Quality of Health Care in America noted that improving our health system depends in very large part on trust. In particular, the IOM indicated that health care professionals must feel that their team members, leaders, and organizations are trustworthy (Institute of Medicine, 2001). Happily, emerging evidence indicates a moderate to high level of trust amongst health care providers (Rushton, Reina, Francovich, Naumann, & Reina, 2010).

Interestingly, the biggest threat to the development and maintenance of trust in a clinical setting is gossip. In fact, the most pervasive behaviors identified as breaking trust included gossip (not speaking with good purpose), breaking confidentiality, and not giving constructive feedback (Rushton et al., 2010).

So what makes us gossip? Traditionally, researchers have thought that rumors spread because of the "Three Cs": conflict, crisis, and catastrophe. But marketing professor Jonah Berger has another idea: What about mere physiological arousal? Berger designed a study in which he placed people into two groups. One group experienced heightened levels of physiological arousal (their autonomic nervous system was activated, which affected bodily functions such as heart rate and perspiration) and the second group did not.

He found that situations that increase arousal spark information sharing—even if the arousal is entirely unrelated to the content of the information being shared (Beilock, 2011; Berger,

2011). That means after you take a jog around the neighborhood, you probably shouldn't stop to chat with your neighbor because you might accidentally spill the beans about your friend's pending divorce. It also means that as a nurse, after you've just participated in a code, you're more likely to mention that piece of office gossip you *had* been keeping to yourself.

One situation that may promote gossip is institutional change. Commentator Donna Kandsberger notes,

> *When communication is not provided until decisions are finalized, unofficial information will certainly spread and fill in any gaps. Typically, due to the anxiety associated with change and unknown outcomes, the scenarios that staff imagine and circulate through the "grapevine" tend to be more negative and alarming than the actual situation.*

Sharing gossip may not always be a bad thing, however. It turns out that there is more than one type of gossip. In fact, authors distinguish between what they call "positive gossip" and "negative gossip" (the latter sometimes referred to colloquially as "trash talk"). When you think about it, people really do spend a lot of time—the majority of their speaking time, according to some studies—talking about other people. Some authors define gossip *very* broadly as the positive or negative information exchange about an absent third party. Using this definition, some gossip may actually be constructive, such as when one coworker tells another coworker that a third party was really helpful during a busy shift (Grosser, Lopez-Kidwell, & Labianca, 2010). But of course, the bottom line is that when most folks think of gossip, they think of the *negative* exchange of sometimes-false information about someone else.

Gossip and verbal abuse may also serve some sociological function—specifically, to help members of a group bond. In a health care setting, there are clearly a number of opposing groups: nurses versus physicians, day shift versus night shift, leadership versus bedside nurses, full-time versus part-time, men versus women, junior versus experienced—the list goes on. Gossip can occur between groups—where, for example, workers on the day shift gossip about those on the night shift. Or, it can happen within groups—for example, one bedside nurse talking about another bedside nurse. The gossip that occurs between groups may serve to reinforce dividing lines that separate one group of people from another. As these battle lines become more entrenched, it can become harder and harder for groups to work together. Although gossiping about someone outside your group with a member of your group can reinforce your group bond, the net effect is negative because it alienates you further from out-of-group colleagues.

What's fascinating is that almost everyone reports experiencing some negative gossip, or peer verbal abuse, at work. Recently, Diane Ceravolo and her colleagues did a study on the frequency of verbal abuse for nurses before and after an intervention workshop series. At baseline, they found—in line with other studies—that 90% of nurses reported experiencing peer verbal abuse in their workplace. After their workshop intervention, the level of verbal abuse decreased to 76%—still quite high.

Sadly, very few (less than one-third) of those affected discussed their experiences with their manager. In fact, nurses reported that talking with their manager about verbal abuse was not effective in resolving the problem (Ceravolo, Schwartz, Foltz-Ramos, & Castner, 2012). This is significant. If the vast majority of nurses experience verbal abuse, and the vast majority also believe that talking with their manager won't help resolve the problem, the obvious question is, what now? What should nurses do when they experience verbal abuse? What should managers do when their nurses report that they have experienced verbal abuse, or that gossip is getting out of control?

Because it doesn't seem realistic to try to change the foundational sociology of human relations by asking employees not to talk about third parties, managers must find another way of dealing with this problem. One approach might be an in-service event to educate nurses about the IOM report on errors, which indicates that many medical mistakes occur due to breakdowns in communication (Institute of Medicine, 1999).

Another might be to maintain an open-door policy so that employees can talk to you easily—and to let them know that the conversation will be treated with respect and not held against them.

If you're dealing with gossip about institutional change, commentator Donna Kansdberger suggests the following:

Initiating communication early along with regular updates can help staff members feel included in the overall goals and mission of the work unit or organization and thus increase their feeling of being respected members of the organization. It must be clearly communicated and understood, in order to avoid the perception of indecision or confusion on the part of the organization's leaders, that early information will be accurate at the time of presentation but is subject to revision over time as plans and decisions evolve. With early and ongoing communication, opportunities for staff to comment or ask questions can increase their feelings of inclusion and empowerment as well as give leaders valuable insights into the "word on the street" or "grapevine" of information and perception that is circulating among the staff.

The bottom line is that it's unlikely that gossip and trash talk is going to vanish from our workplace, so we need to find constructive ways of managing its negative consequences.

Commentator Melissa Snyder articulates three approaches a nurse manager can take to address this type of inappropriate communication:

First, the nurse manager must consistently work at establishing professional relationships among all employees based on trust and integrity. Without these core values, relationships cannot grow and mature, and the cohesiveness of the work team is constantly challenged. In a busy, stressful health care environment, nurses must feel supported by and confident in the abilities of their colleagues. The scenarios in this chapter reveal a betrayal and threat to trust and support in both personal and professional ways.

To establish trust, nurses must be empowered to share their thoughts and feelings regarding situations in a professional way.

The second approach in dealing with gossip and trash talk is to foster a professional work environment that extends beyond the boundaries of a particular unit. Professionalism must be modeled consistently by the nurse manager and other expert nurses. In addition, all nurses should be supported in their socialization to the professional role with frequent opportunities to practice these skills and to gain new knowledge through professional development programs. Over time, this combination creates an expectation of professional behavior that guides how nurses behave at the bedside but also permeates all other aspects of their lives.

The final approach is the need to address the role of technology and social media with all nurses. Nurses need to know that these technologies can be very useful but can also be very detrimental if not used with caution and consideration. Nurses need to know what the expectations are for their use of social media, and if possible there should be a clear policy indicating how these technologies can be used.

Vignettes, Commentaries, and Reflective Thinking

The remainder of this chapter presents vignettes about gossip and trash talking, commentaries about the experiences represented in the vignettes, and opportunities to explore or reflect on the material.

Vignette 3.1: Indiscretion

Liz is an OR nurse known for her love of "sharing" information about her coworkers. During her shift, she often goes from one nurse to the next, prompting them with "Did you know…?" or "Have you heard the latest?"

Most of the other nurses know what Liz is up to and have learned to deflect her. Even so, her constant desire to spread negative news creates friction in the OR—especially when Liz repeats information about one nurse to another. She is a master at taking tidbits of conversations out of context and sharing them with a person they are likely to upset.

Penny, an OR tech, is good buddies with Liz and often collaborates with her to spread rumors. Between the two of them, Liz and Penny stir up lots of drama in the OR. One day, Liz and Penny suggest that Tara, a nurse who has been having marital trouble, has filed for divorce from her abusive husband. Within hours, everyone in the OR thinks that Tara's marriage is on the rocks, and, when one nurse comes up to console her, Tara becomes upset. She goes to the manager and insists that something be done to curtail Liz and Penny's "loose lips."

Expert Commentary: Vignette 3.1

The manager of the OR needs to go directly to the source of the rumor mill and confront both Liz and Penny about their actions. It is possible that the pair may find this to be a harmless activity or that they are really unaware of the way their actions are affecting others. This direct confrontation may be enough to curtail their desire to share rumors—especially if they are informed of the negative effects this behavior is having on other staff members.

Sometimes, simply recognizing the problem is enough incentive to end the behavior. However, the manager might decide to speak with the staff as a whole. In this exchange, the staff could be empowered to speak up when they are uncomfortable with information that is being shared by their colleagues.

Without a willing audience, the rumors cannot be spread—and this may be the most effective way of resolving the problem. In a unit such as the OR, where everyone must work together as an orchestrated team, integrity and trust are core values that are essential to building a cohesive work group. The rumor mill whittles away at the integrity of all who participate in this activity. Over time, it will affect the ability of the group to function as a unified staff.

—Melissa Snyder

Just as with younger girls, those who control the flow of information often perceive themselves as having a sense of power. Knowing the latest tidbits about classmates or coworkers and selectively sharing them (or not) can seem to bestow status and even popularity, but this tactic may misfire.

As a manager, I would engage the entire OR staff in some way to raise awareness about the separation between personal and professional lives. Yes, it's nice to have colleagues who care about you and your well-being, but the place to address those concerns is almost always face to face—*not* through an intermediary or third party. Depending on the severity of the problem, there might need to be a more systematic ongoing program to educate everyone on respect and civility.

Distortion of information can also lead to serious misunderstandings about important topics. At a staff meeting, I would want everyone to use more caution in what they share about coworkers; the OR is a small community in and of itself where rumors can fly quickly. At the same time, I would indicate my approval of those nurses who use discretion and understand that when something comes their way, it should be kept confidential or at least not shared more widely.

Lastly, I would have a conversation with Liz and Penny individually to try to gauge their time management, their job performance, and their professional development. If loose lips are causing problems with work, they need feedback on that. As well, given Liz and Penny's ability to share information, I might invite them to develop a newsletter or some other form of communication to be shared by all OR personnel.

—Cheryl Dellasega

Reflection

Do certain nurses in your unit share personal information about coworkers with third parties? Do *you*? If you're being honest, the answer to this question is "yes." It's normal to talk about our friends and colleagues; the problem arises when we're malicious or cruel.

One critical question to consider is whether the gossip is disruptive to the unit's cohesion. The question then becomes: what can you as the nurse manager do about it?

Vignette 3.2: Out of Context

One busy evening, Liandra—who has worked in the ED for many years—makes a medication error, which is quickly caught and corrected by one of her coworkers. Despite the self-limiting nature of the medication mistake, Liandra is consumed with guilt. She can't stop retracing her steps and trying to figure out what led her to give the wrong dose of medication.

Carrie, Liandra's coworker, works a double on the night after the mistake is made. She tells the entire night shift about Liandra, implying that the nurse manager is ready to take further action. By morning, the night shift workers are convinced Liandra nearly killed a patient and will suffer serious repercussions.

One of them calls Liandra to console her and discovers the incident has been blown out of proportion. This is not the first time Carrie has been caught exaggerating at the expense of a coworker.

Expert Commentary: Vignette 3.2

When things go wrong within a clinical setting, it is important to have established a culture in which the error is reported rapidly and the focus is not on blaming the person who made the error, but on exploring why the error occurred and preventing future errors. In this vignette, Carrie has created a culture of blame through her exaggeration of the error made by Liandra.

The focus is now on correcting the misinformation and negative feeling created by this exaggeration. As the manager, it would be important to directly address this issue with Carrie and help her understand how her actions have created an environment that is not only problematic for her colleagues but also shifts the focus from prevention of these errors to seeking blame for an error that anyone could make—again. The manager should work with the staff to create a culture of trust that encourages the staff to report errors quickly and accurately without fear of repercussions from other staff. And when errors like the one in this vignette occur, the approach can be changed so as to seek opportunities for new learning at all levels.

–Melissa Snyder

My first concern in this situation would be Liandra's well-being—assuming, of course, that the patient has been taken care of. I would act quickly to address the situation by reinforcing the process to be followed when mistakes are made, stressing that patient safety comes first. With Liandra, I would try to identify factors that may have contributed to the mistake in case system issues need to be corrected.

Next, I would have a unit-wide discussion on errors. This would provide an opportunity for all ED personnel to discuss how we as professionals address mistakes. It would be helpful if others volunteered ahead of time to share incidents in which they have made errors and how they dealt with both the ethical and emotional aspects. This might be the venue to further examine the damage done when negative talk occurs around a coworker's performance.

Finally, I would want to check back with Liandra and make sure her professional self-esteem is back on track. If she continues to feel guilty and unsure of herself, the likelihood of future mistakes will increase. Other senior nurses could also be encouraged to be supportive of Liandra and check in with her from time to time.

–Cheryl Dellasega

Reflection

Most of us played the game "telephone" as kids, where a message begins with one person and is slowly—and reliably—distorted as it makes its way from one person to the next. As the nurse manager, what can you do when this type of thing happens on your unit? If gossip is just part of human nature—and we won't be able to eliminate it—what can we do to contsructively manage it?

In the case above, Liandra makes a mistake. When errors occur on your unit, how does the staff react? Does the person who made the error feel free to report it? Are others in the unit emotionally supportive of the nurse who made the error? In short: What type of environment has been cultivated on your unit? Are you satisfied with it?

Vignette 3.3: Secrets

For several months, Maggie has been trying to get pregnant. She and her husband, a resident in the same hospital where she works, have gone through several special treatments to try and have a child. When she finally conceives, she tells only Alice, another nurse supervisor with whom she is close.

"Please keep it to yourself," Maggie says. "I'm worried something might go wrong, and anyway, I'm applying for that new position in nursing education. If they know I'm pregnant, I might not get the job."

Alice tells Maggie she will keep her secret, but over coffee with Donna, she hints about some big news that is about to break. Donna, who knows Maggie, guesses at the secret, which Alice refuses to confirm with anything more than a smile. Donna then progresses to tell two other people who "promise" not to reveal what they know, and so on. Eventually, Maggie learns about Alice's betrayal and confronts her—so angry that the relationship is permanently damaged.

Expert Commentary: Vignette 3.3

In this vignette, Maggie has not directly contacted the nurse manager. However, it is safe to assume that the nurse manager will be aware of the issue through other staff. At this point, the manager must address this issue with both Maggie and Alice. Because Maggie is angry and feeling betrayed, these emotions must be addressed. It is also important for Maggie and Alice to meet to discuss the situation.

Maggie may need some coaching to help her manage her intense feelings of anger and betrayal, while Alice needs coaching regarding her inability to keep information in confidence. Working on ways to reestablish trust is imperative not only to maintaining the relationship between the two nurses, but also to maintaining the integrity of the unit as a functioning whole. The manager's role is not to get involved in the personal relationships of the staff, but to assist all staff in maintaining relationships that are professional and support the overall workings of the unit.

Assisting staff in recognizing the difference between professional and nonprofessional communication is crucial and must be reinforced in circumstances like this one. It is important for the manager to help Alice understand that this indiscretion makes others question her ability to keep information confidential. Confidentiality is essential in health care settings.

–Melissa Snyder

This situation provides a good opportunity to apply rules protecting patient privacy to standards we set for coworkers. If the facts of this situation were slightly different, Alice would have violated HIPAA laws about privacy of information.

Respecting a person's request for confidentiality is part of a trust relationship, and trust is integral to teamwork. Team-building and morale activities can help everyone move forward with a better understanding of ways to support and respect each other.

The influence of body language as part of communication is important. Something as subtle as rolling your eyes or sighing loudly can turn a neutral message negative.

If the opportunity presented itself, I might also have a conversation with Alice and/or Maggie to see whether the relationship between them can be repaired. There's no way to undo the damage, but it might be possible to forgive and move on.

–Cheryl Dellasega

Reflection

Good news is hard to keep to yourself. Sometimes when we gossip, it's not necessarily malicious—we're just so excited to be part of something new, fun, and exciting that the words tumble from our lips. The problem, of course, is that this type of behavior can cause serious dysfunction. Have you ever experienced a similar situation? Was there fallout in your unit? What did you do to address it?

Vignette 3.4: Cyberbullying

Kim, a young, attractive, unmarried nurse, is the hub of social activities on the step-down unit (SDU). She often organizes parties and other after-work activities.

A competition starts between Kim and Nora, another nurse, when they both become romantically interested in Matt, a second-year resident. When Kim sees Nora openly flirting with Matt after he has made rounds, she is furious. Later, Kim uses her cell phone to take an unflattering picture of Nora from the rear. That evening, she posts the picture on Facebook with the comment: "Someone needs to diet—NOW!"

When Nora sees the picture, Kim shrugs it off and says it was a joke. Nora doesn't find it funny and threatens to go to human resources over the incident.

Expert Commentary: Vignette 3.4

Cyberbullying is a very real concern and should be taken seriously by all nurses and nurse managers. In this situation, the nurse manager should directly address the issue with Kim. Kim needs to be aware that her actions are unprofessional. Even though the comments and the Facebook picture are not related to work activities, they reflect poorly on her professional character.

Managers can encourage social activities among staff members. These activities help to build camaraderie and can help with stress management. However, it is essential to remember that professional behavior is required even in these situations.

It is important for nurses to be reminded that social media is a tool that needs to be managed very carefully. On social media, nurses must consistently reflect an image that is not in conflict with their professional role. If there is any question about the content, it should not be posted. Keep in mind that if you would not share something directly in a face-to-face interaction, it should not be shared on social media.

Additionally, the flirting behaviors are also problematic and need to be addressed by the nurse manager. These behaviors are also unprofessional and inappropriate during work time. Maintaining a professional demeanor in all interpersonal interactions is required. Any behavior that does not meet this standard should be addressed.

–Melissa Snyder

Posting unflattering pictures and/or videos is the most severe form of cyberbullying for adults. Knowing this, a policy about what is and is not posted about coworkers can be put in place. As a nurse manager, I can't control what goes on in an individual's personal life. I can, however, set expectations for professionalism in the workplace. Sharing exemplars (examples that are not likely to identify anyone on your unit or violate confidentiality of others) could start a dialogue on each person's comfort zone when it comes to social media. It might not hurt to have someone from human resources or the legal department come in and discuss other potential consequences of sharing material online without express permission from everyone involved.

Kim is clearly in the wrong, so I would want to have a conversation with her first. Then I would bring Kim and Nora in together to reconcile the situation. Techniques for restorative justice can possibly help the two of them work through their feelings of anger and hurt (http://www.restorativejustice.org/). Finally, I would observe Matt's behavior as well, since males have been known to fan the flames of jealous rivalry between two potential romantic interests. Making it clear that drama over a perceived flirtation during work time is not acceptable would be another priority, but that conversation might have to occur more informally. Certainly, if the opportunity to talk to the residency director about Matt's behavior arose, I would definitely fill him/her in.

–Cheryl Dellasega

Reflection

Is flirting a common behavior on your unit? Is it wrong to flirt at work? Why? If it *is* wrong, how might you, as the nurse manager, address it?

If an event like the one described in this vignette occurred on your unit, how would you respond? Do you think Kim could be fired over the incident? How would you try to get these two to work together?

Vignette 3.5: Rumors

Tanya, an RN in the ED, is on break during a slightly slow day shift. She decides to catch up on texts. While composing a message to Dean, a nurse on the evening shift, she gets a call and stops to respond to it.

The caller is Sonya, who wants to share some news with Tanya: Susan, the ED nurse manager, is going to be "replaced" by the end of the week. Tanya has had a rocky relationship with Susan, so she considers this good news and can't wait to text Dean. As soon as she stops talking to Sonya, she texts Dean: "Guess what? That b---- Susan is going to be fired!"

Accidentally, Tanya sends the text to Deandra, who is one of Susan's best friends. Deandra instantly contacts Susan, and learns that Susan is, in fact, being promoted and another nurse manager designated.

Expert Commentary: Vignette 3.5

In this situation, Tanya's behavior is extremely unprofessional. Two key issues seem to be occurring simultaneously within this vignette. First, the use of technology in communicating information must be addressed. Within a matter of minutes, Tanya has managed to involve four other nurses in her unprofessional and inaccurate communication. The second issue involves the derogatory terms used in sharing the information about a colleague.

With regard to the first issue, as the nurse manager, it is important to discuss professional and unprofessional communications both in person and via technology. The most critical message is the need to confirm the accuracy of all information before sending it forward via technology. Because of the speed of communication, inaccurate information can be distributed to known and unknown sources within seconds—and it cannot be easily corrected when new information emerges. Tanya must be reminded of this. It is also important to discuss this issue with the entire staff so that everyone recognizes the power and the detriments of communicating through technology.

With regard to the second issue, this language is unprofessional and disrespectful. Even though the message was intended to be a personal communication, it quickly became a more public message. Tanya's professional reputation is in jeopardy, and a sincere apology by Tanya to all involved individuals is necessary. The nurse manager will be the one to directly address this issue with Tanya and recommend that Tanya apologize for her actions as a first step to rebuilding a professional relationship with Susan and Deandra. Again, discussing the very gray area between personal and professional communications is important. Nurses need to be encouraged to always err on the side of caution, especially when sharing information that may have an effect on others.

–Melissa Snyder

Technology can hurt as much as it helps. Many helpful applications can simplify our lives, but the rapid pace of conversations can also lead to messages with inflammatory content being sent to the wrong person. In this situation, Tanya clearly made a mistake, and the sooner she apologizes, the better.

Because this issue occurred during work, it's a good opportunity to discuss acceptable downtime activities. Establishing a policy for use of personal cell phones and other technologies during work time can prevent more problems with this behavior, but the guidelines would have to be very explicit and consequences for violations clear.

On a higher level, this situation presents an opportunity to address what is likely to be an institution-wide challenge. If other administrators are willing to cooperate and create a policy that will apply to every employee, the intervention will be more powerful. There might be a need to collect data on other types of tech issues that can also be addressed by administrative leaders.

–Cheryl Dellasega

Reflection

Obviously, there's a lot that's less than ideal about Tanya's behavior. On a broad level: What institutional/unit culture do you think made Tanya comfortable (1) texting at work, (2) calling a colleague a b---- at work, and (3) spreading untrue gossip? Do any of *your* behaviors perpetuate that culture? If so, what can you do about it?

On a narrower level: If a nurse on your unit ever sent an inflammatory text or email to the wrong person in error, what action would you take? Does your organization have a policy on the use of cell phones during work hours? If not, should it?

Summary

Gossip is a fundamental part of human behavior. We gossip at home; we gossip at work; we gossip everywhere! It's not always bad: Sometimes we gossip because we're so excited to share some good news or to say a kind word about someone else. Often, though, we gossip with malicous intent. We say things that aren't true—things that are exaggerated or unkind.

Gossip and negative trash talk can take on a life of their own, poisoning a unit and spilling into other venues such as home and leisure activities. Often, the consequences of gossip aren't clearly understood nor are the ways to address it.

Given that it's unlikely we can change human behavior, we need to establish strategies for (1) reducing negative gossip and (2) dealing with it when it happens. Education is always a good place to start. Education that takes the form of an open conversation is also often helpful—that way nurses feel that their voice is being heard. And—of critical importance—nurse managers must model the professional behavior they want to see. If you as the nurse manager gossip, how can you really ask your nurses to stop?

The nurse manager is a role model who provides an example of desired behavior. Monitor your own interactions and make sure you aren't inadvertently passing along bits of information that may or may not be true. Challenge your staff to adopt a zero-tolerance policy for gossip—start with one shift, then see if you can increase to 1 day, 1 week, 1 month, and so on. Once the cycle of negative interations is changed, the work environment will be more enjoyable for everyone involved. Use the activities below to further work on decreasing gossip and other caustic conversation.

Activities

"Sharon told Millie that Carrie, a coworker, seemed withdrawn lately and was seeing a psychiatrist. In turn, Millie expressed concern about Carrie's well-being to four other coworkers they both knew, and they shared the information with four more. Before long, Carrie's depression was common knowledge in the small organization where she worked—except that Carrie wasn't depressed. She was dating a psychiatrist, which is why she was seen entering his office during her day off."

Ask staff (or yourself) to use the "Gossip Filter" test to answer these four questions:

- Did Millie receive the information shared firsthand?

- Did Millie know for a fact that the information was true?

- What was Millie's motivation for sharing the information?

- Would Millie have shared the same information if Carrie was present?

Next, ask everyone to think about a recent incident where some spicy information or potential gossip came their way, and use the four questions above to evaluate the situation and whether the information was shared or not. Encourage use of the "Gossip Filter" in the future.

Alternatively, discuss how you can reduce gossip and brainstorm strategies for holding yourself and others accountable. Create a poster or other reminder that caring doesn't always mean sharing information that could be harmful to another.

4 | cliques, campaigns, and high-school drama

Nurses describe a variety of behaviors that teen girls often call "drama." There are "campaigns," where a group of nurses targets a coworker, ganging up on him or her so he or she becomes a persona non grata. There are drama queens who deliberately create trouble and discord. There are those who display "two-faced" behavior—i.e., the nurse acts sweet when managers are around and sinister when they are gone. Even patient assignments can be used as a weapon to punish individual nurses.

Townsend (2012) describes the "bullying culture" of the nursing profession and its adverse impact on health status, patient care, and finances. She states that most nurses have witnessed this behavior, and that nurse managers are the ones who can break the cycle and create a new culture. Her advice: "Nurse managers should encourage staff to report bullying incidents, ensure that those who experience and report abusive incidents will be safe from retribution, and take action to discipline bullies, counsel victims, and implement corrective measures to prevent recurrence. Bullying can be addressed by unit-based councils, with council members serving as role models for other staff members" (Creating a healthy work environment, para. 3). Also, a zero-tolerance policy is helpful.

A nurse manager who commented on Townsend's article wrote the following:

> *Love that the managers are being bashed here and for good reason. The manager sets the tone in any environment. I*

am proud to say that through my zero-tolerance policy I got rid of the bullies in my units when I started 4 years ago. Step up or step out—not hard. For those of you who are staff nurses, my advice, document everything and continue to report it. [Bullying] is being looked at on the federal level as a workplace issue like discrimination so there is hope that things will change. (Townsend, 2012, Comments, para.11).

Sandra Barton and her colleagues (2011) describe the exclusion that occurs within health care, stating that "Managers must recognize whether their staff is working as a team or as a clique." They believe nursing cliques have a negative impact on retention and lead to adverse physical symptoms in employees. Because retention rates, absenteeism, and cost figures are used to evaluate the performance of nurse managers, the impact of cliques may have a personal repercussion. They advise not blaming, promoting teamwork, good communication skills, and celebrating differences.

Hutchinson, Jackson, Wilkes, and Vickers (2008) presented an elegant analysis of bullying that expresses what nurses post about and often tell us. They are the first to describe organizational aspects (informal organizational alliances, formal and informal reward systems, misuse of authority) as antecedents of bullying, which manifest initially as personal attacks, then an attack on work product, and finally an attack on reputation and competence.

A bullied nurse often develops a perceived failure or flaw as both an employee and a person in response to abuse. Hutchinson and colleagues say that the process just described often leads to stigmatization of the nurse as incompetent. They, too, describe a normalization of bullying that occurs because of a lack of accountability and a tolerance of bullying, because these individuals are often high performers. Indeed, they may even be the ones who get promoted. They assert that while policies may be in place, informal alliances prevent them from being fully implemented, often because the nurse manager is a bully.

Susan Johnson, one of our commentators, believes that nurse managers need to check in with all parties in situations of conflict, including witnesses, before taking action, because bullies can retaliate against people who report their behavior. This creates a situation in which people are reluctant to bring forth further complaints due to fear. Furthermore, when bullying behaviors include criticizing the clinical competency of others, targets are often reluctant to report this to managers, because they are afraid they will be disciplined or fired for poor performance. If there are clinical performance issues, managers are in a position to deal with these; however, they also need to make sure that they deal with the behavioral issues as well (such as publicly criticizing the performance of another nurse).

Mary Johansen (2012) suggests that nurse managers use the following strategies to keep the peace:

- Clarifying what constitutes conflict

- Being aware of your conflict-management style (see Appendix A, "Is Your Management Style Causing Conflict?")

- Avoiding a perception of punishment

- Initiating dialogue

- Being a coach

- Discussing conflicts proactively

- Raising awareness and ability through education and training

Johansen provides a case scenario and evaluation that can be useful for raising awareness and ability. Should you want to use this approach, a case scenario for this purpose is contained in Appendix B, "Conflict Case Scenario."

Vignettes, Commentaries, and Reflective Thinking

The remainder of this chapter presents vignettes about cliques, campaigns, and high-school drama, commentaries about the experiences represented in the vignettes, and opportunities to explore or reflect on the material.

Vignette 4.1: Ganging Up

Mia is the unit secretary on a busy surgical unit staffed with both LPNs and RNs. She takes a dislike to Gretchen, a newer RN who is working on her graduate degree in education and who Mia thinks is "uppity."

"My class assignment this week is really hard," Gretchen says to an RN coworker, within earshot of Mia. "You really have to be in the swing of school to stay on top of things like this."

Mia waits until she is alone with Vicky, one of the unit LPNs. "You know, that Gretchen is really full of herself," Mia tells Vicky. "I heard her talking the other day about how well educated she is and how only people who are real scholars can go to college."

Vicky, who constantly worries the hospital will phase out LPNs, is instantly disturbed by Mia's revelation. She tells the other LPN coworkers that the RNs think they are better than LPNs, and an all-out word war begins. At the heart of it is Gretchen, who receives no LPN help with her patients and is targeted by both the LPNs and, eventually, the RNs, who begin to believe she was insulting their educational preparation as well.

Expert Commentary: Vignette 4.1

In this scenario, there are several behaviors that are inappropriate: gossiping, maligning the personal reputation of another worker, and refusing to help another worker. The behavioral issues cannot be pinned on one person, however. Unit-level intervention is needed.

The first step would be to provide a mandatory in-service on workplace bullying and incivility. The focus of this would be to educate staff about what types of behaviors are inappropriate. If there are any pertinent organization-wide policies that address this behavior, they need to be discussed in the in-service and posted in the unit.

The second step would be to craft a unit-specific code of conduct that addresses acceptable and unacceptable behaviors. All staff should have an opportunity to contribute to the drafting of this code of conduct, but managers should make sure that the specific disruptive behaviors they are currently experiencing are included. After the code of conduct has been drafted, everyone should sign it, and it should be posted in a prominent area. Individual copies should also be distributed. In addition, new staff members should be asked to sign the code when they come on, and all staff members should renew their commitment to the code on a yearly basis.

The code of conduct can be used by both managers and staff to call out incidences of undesirable behaviors as they happen. It can also be used by managers if they need to engage in informal or formal discussions with staff regarding behavioral issues. The manager also needs to follow up with Gretchen to make sure the problem is resolved and that she is getting the assistance she needs from the other staff.

–Susan Johnson

This is a tough situation. The nurse manager has to be sensitive to the gossip that's flying around and figure out how all this started. She needs to be frank and put her cards on the table to put a stop to the bad talk quickly. Everyone has to tell the truth so the nurse manager can trace the source of the rumors. Negative gossip can be infectious and permeate everything. If coworkers behave this way, it puts patients at risk, because there are different groups and one won't help another out of spite.

First, hold a general meeting to figure out who is at the source of the word war. Then follow-up with that person one-on-one to tell him or her such behavior won't be tolerated. It's too disruptive. This situation was disrespectful to both RNs and LPNs. The unit secretary deliberately pitted one person against the other.

This is not easy, but it is a situation in which the RNs and LPNs must come together and the nurse manager must say: "Apparently there's a general feeling that RNs are better because they are more educated. All of us bring certain things to the table, and everyone learns from everyone else. If you haven't learned something today, you haven't been paying attention."

That discussion doesn't mean one person is better or worse. Nurses have to stay focused on the fact that the patient is the center of what they are doing, so they can work together for his or her benefit. This needs to be an up-front conversation, and people need to be held accountable.

–Kathy Curci

Reflection

Do nurses on your unit develop cliques and engage in campaigns? Are nurses in your unit divided—RNs versus LPNs? What behaviors occur as a consequence of this division?

Do nurses with lower degrees feel threatened by nurses who have pursued or are pursuing additional education?

Are there certain nurses on your unit who refuse to help their colleagues out because of interpersonal conflict, as with Gretchen? If so, what can you do about it?

Vignette 4.2: Witness

Day after day, Priscilla watches Melissa, the evening shift full-timer, bully her coworkers. She is bossy and insulting to other nurses, but especially to Amanda, the day-shift nurse who usually reports off to her.

"Make sure you get your facts straight," she tells Amanda in front of a crowd of their coworkers. "Yesterday I checked on the IV you said was fine and it wasn't. The site was red and clearly infected, so now that patient is very uncomfortable."

"Are you saying I did something to deliberately hurt a patient?" Amanda asks.

"Yes, pretty much," Melissa snaps back. "You're in charge of an accurate report, so if you tell me something that clearly couldn't have been true, you're responsible."

Amanda pauses for a moment to collect herself, clearly upset, while Melissa grabs the medication cart and stalks off down the hallway.

Expert Commentary: Vignette 4.2

The main issue in this scenario is that Melissa is giving inappropriate feedback to Amanda. If there are issues that affect patient care, she needs to discuss them with Amanda privately or ask management to address the issues. It is never appropriate to give feedback regarding patient care in a public manner.

There are several actions that Priscilla can take in this scenario. She can first check with Amanda to see how she feels about the situation and whether she has discussed it with Melissa or her manager. If the two feel comfortable, their next step might then be to discuss the issue with Melissa. If they take this step and the behavior doesn't change, they need to talk with their manager. Similarly, they should talk to their manager right away if they feel talking with Melissa will escalate the situation or lead to retaliation. Priscilla can offer to go with Amanda when she talks with the manager to provide moral support and corroboration of Amanda's story.

Both Amanda and Priscilla should be willing to document any complaints they have. The manager needs to let Melissa know her current behavior is inappropriate and take the initiative to set expectations for future behavior. The manager needs to follow up with Amanda, Priscilla, and Melissa on a regular basis to make sure the behavioral changes are being made.

–Susan Johnson

Amanda needs to stand up to Melissa and say, "You will not talk to me like this, period." If Amanda can't do it alone, she needs to have the nurse manager there for support. It's hard to believe Melissa treats only Amanda this way. It's more likely that for her whole career, she has treated coworkers in this manner.

Melissa comes off as not a very nice person. It's hard as a new nurse to stand up to someone who's been there a long time, but frame it as having respect for yourself. If someone is upset with a nurse, the nurse needs to tell the person, "You know what? If I'm not doing something right, I want to learn from it."

Melissa is not being helpful in her feedback to Amanda. The bullying behavior isn't likely to be corrected in one conversation, but it needs to be addressed with the aggressive nurse. If a new nurse can't do it alone, the nurse manager has a responsibility to make sure Melissa and all nurses treat everyone—coworkers and patients—with respect. If a nurse can't be a team player, then he or she is going to have to go play somewhere else.

–Kathy Curci

Reflection

What do you think is going on in Melissa's life that creates the need to "dress down" other nurses in public? Is it possible that the culture of your unit makes Melissa feel like it's OK to engage in this type of behavior? What are some steps you—the nurse manager—can take to try to adjust the culture of your unit?

Vignette 4.3: Energy Vampire

Hilary is a part-time float nurse on the pediatric unit, where critically ill children come and go quickly. Since she first began work 2 years ago, Hilary has been "high maintenance" for the other nurses—she expects them to treat her differently. "I'm just a part-timer," she frequently points out. "I can't keep up with all these policies and procedures."

One morning Hilary calls her nurse manager, Becca, after working the previous evening shift. "Everyone on evenings is so mean," she sobs. "They just kept criticizing me all evening."

When Becca checks with evening-shift nurses, she finds out that Hilary demanded a great deal of attention and created drama when she didn't get her way. Two days later, the scenario repeats itself when Hilary is assigned to help out in the pediatric ICU. "Never send her again," Carol, a PICU nurse, tells Becca. "I'd rather be shot than deal with her. She takes more energy than it's worth."

Expert Commentary: Vignette 4.3

In this scenario, the manager needs to create a performance plan for Hilary. One of the expectations is that Hilary will keep abreast of unit standards, policies, and procedures. The manager could also set expectations that Hilary will comport herself in a professional manner—which means no dramatic outbursts at the nurses' station. Staff members need to be encouraged to help Hilary if appropriate, but they should also document incidences when she is not meeting performance standards. Instead of criticizing Hillary or her performance publicly, invite staff to bring concerns to the attention of management, which will then address the issues. Management should have periodic meetings with Hilary and the charge nurse on the evening shift to determine whether Hilary's behavior is changing.

Managers can never assume that they are hearing the whole story from one party. The person reporting the behavior may be incorrectly assessing the situation or purposely trying to get someone else in trouble. Whenever managers take action against inappropriate behaviors in the workplace, follow-up with the target of the behavior, the perpetrator of the behavior, and coworkers is needed. Managers can't assume that behavior has changed just because staff does not continue to report it. Staff may wrongly assume that if behaviors do not change, it is because management cannot or will not do anything about them.

–Susan Johnson

The expectation is that when you're a float nurse, you're assigned to places where they are short staffed. A float nurse needs to be able to step in and do the job. If the float nurse can't keep up with the policies and procedures, he or she needs to learn them. It's not the coworkers' responsibility to hold his or her hand. In terms of patient care, the expectations of a float nurse are the same as for anyone else.

Becca can tell Hilary that people aren't "being mean" to her; they're just frustrated. They're short staffed and end up having to help her instead of vice versa. Hilary may realize she needs to become more informed about policies or step up to the plate in some other way. If she can't, she needs to go back to Becca and ask for more orientation and time.

From that point on, Becca is responsible for providing what Hilary needs, but if Hilary doesn't tell her, Becca won't know. Everything will continue—Hilary will feel picked on, and everyone else will feel frustrated. But Hilary has to be mature enough to admit to her limitations and take measures to address them. Becca must take responsibility as a nurse manager who supports her nurses and wants to see them satisfied and fulfilled by their work.

–Kathy Curci

Reflection

Your hospital may have part-time, temporary, or float nurses. Does your staff find it harder to work with nurses who are not a permanent part of their unit? Why or why not? How do you greet new nurses who come to work on your unit on a short-term basis?

Do you think it's harder to *be* a float nurse? Why might a nurse choose to float? What do you think are the strengths and limitations—in general—of a nurse who chooses to be a float nurse? How can you work around those pros and cons?

Vignette 4.4: Two-Faced

Two of the nurses on the MICU day shift are notorious for acting one way when management nurses are around, and another when they're gone. Dana and Bonnie, longtimers on the unit, know when the nurse manager is likely to show up and make a point of acting superbusy and supercordial when that occurs. As soon as the nurse manager leaves the unit, they slack off and hide out in the breakroom, gossiping, while Nadine, a newer nurse, picks up the slack.

When Nadine asks Dana and Bonnie for help, they only comply if a nurse manager is nearby to see it. Nadine feels "trapped," because Dana and Bonnie will support each other if confronted, and the manager only sees them when they're on "good behavior."

Expert Commentary: Vignette 4.4

Nurse managers can do several things in this scenario. They can talk with others on the unit to get their perceptions of Dana and Bonnie's behaviors. If several witnesses can confirm Nadine's story, they can bring this to Dana and Bonnie's attention and come up with a plan for changing their behavior. If Nadine is the only one who reports the behavior, management needs to show up on the unit at times when they are not expected and make their own observations. Management can instruct Nadine to stop picking up the slack for Dana and Bonnie, so they become responsible for their own work. If Nadine stops covering for Dana and Bonnie, then management can hold them accountable for work they are not doing.

–Susan Johnson

Nadine needs to privately meet with the nurse manager and share what's happening, but not in a tattletale way. Avoiding accusations, Nadine can just say this is what she is feeling and seeing. She should share her perceptions but expect the nurse manager to validate them by observing Bonnie and Dana when they are not aware she is there.

The nurse manager needs to be ready to help find out what Nadine is feeling. Nadine can help the nurse manager by asking him or her to figure out a way to observe Dana and Bonnie's behavior. Then, based on what the nurse manager finds, he or she knows how to intervene. The expectation is that the behavior would be corrected (assuming Nadine's perceptions are accurate).

It takes a real level of maturity on Nadine's part to handle this well. She may or may not be able to do this without appearing as though she is complaining. The key for nurses is to enlist their nurse manager's help because they don't want to feel frustrated with their work or feel like they aren't part of a team. It takes maturity to spin it right. Anyone is a situation like this would feel it was just not fair, but there's nothing a nurse manager can work with if it's expressed as a complaint. "Help me understand if what I'm feeling is really happening," is a statement that can work.

–Kathy Curci

Reflection

Do you think that your nurses ever put on an act to try to impress you? If so, what can you do about it? Would visiting the floor of your unit at varying times help?

If you believed that a nurse was putting on a show for your benefit, what would you do about it? Would you say something to the nurse? What would you say? How would you say it?

Vignette 4.5: Green-Eyed Monster

Kirstin has moved to the city and started a job in the NICU, where nurses and physicians are on a first-name basis and relationships are more relaxed. As a younger, attractive nurse, Kirstin garners attention from the male physicians. She enjoys this attention and even begins to socialize with some of the residents after work hours.

Kirstin is competent and professional in her patient care, and the previous work she did in a neuro unit gives her a strong background for work in the NICU. The other nurses, however, resent the excitement Kirstin's arrival has caused and the attention she receives from their medical colleagues.

"You wouldn't find me going out for drinks with them after work," comments Fran, an older nurse. Soon, Fran and the other nurses ostracize Kirstin and refuse to help her because her first loyalty seems to be toward the physicians.

Expert Commentary: Vignette 4.5

This is another scenario where a unit-wide intervention in the form of education and a code of conduct would be appropriate. It is not acceptable for the nurses to gossip about conduct that occurs outside of the work environment. As long as the relationships between Kirstin and the physicians are kept on a professional basis during work hours, they are not the concern of anyone at work. Also, it is never appropriate for a nurse to refuse to help another because he or she holds a grudge against that nurse. The code of conduct could also address flirting and other inappropriate action within the workplace to make sure that Kirstin's behavior at work does not become unprofessional. Again, the managers should check back frequently with all parties to make sure these interventions address the issues.

–Susan Johnson

This scenario is happening outside the workplace. It's important to realize that if Kirstin is a good nurse, there's nothing the nurse manager can do. If there's jealousy, she can't get involved or let what's happening outside the hospital affect the work arena. The nurse manager could, however, continue to treat everyone professionally and to stress that what Kirstin does outside of work is her own business—as long as it doesn't affect patients.

If the other nurses refuse to help Kirstin and mistreat her, then the nurse manager can step in and stress the importance of teamwork. What any nurse does outside the unit shouldn't affect his or her work.

No one is asking a nurse to approve of what goes on in a coworker's life after hours. His or her job is to be a good colleague and team member. Nurses need to treat each other with respect and have the attitude that everyone works together. You don't have to agree about their politics or their behavior outside of work, but you do have to work with them to take care of patients.

–Kathy Curci

Reflection

Is Kirstin's behavior unprofessional? Do any of the nurses on your unit see colleagues of the opposite gender outside of work hours? Do you disapprove? If so, why?

If some of the nurses on your unit garner the interest of male colleagues, does it upset the balance of the unit? As the nurse manager, how might you handle this situation?

Vignette 4.6: Who Gets Whom

Linda's first job out of nursing school is at a private, for-profit hospital in Southern California. She likes her job, but after a while, she starts to notice that her patient load is harder than most.

Linda talks with Jane, another new-grad nurse, and says, "I would come in a few minutes before my shift began and discover that my patient load was way, *way* harder than that of my colleagues." Jane and Linda eventually realize that the experienced nurses are coming in for the shift early and switching around the patient load, intentionally giving the nurses who came in later the harder patients.

Jane is trying to give her colleagues the benefit of the doubt and tells Linda that she doesn't think the senior nurses are intentionally trying to be cruel. Linda's perspective is less rosy. She replies, "Maybe not, but they totally know they're screwing *someone* over, making their day way harder." Linda goes on to say, "It's especially inconsiderate because I'm a new graduate, and they should have been helping me, not taking advantage of my ignorance and naiveté! I think what really upsets me is that they don't feel any allegiance to the team at all. They are just looking out for themselves."

Expert Commentary: Vignette 4.6

Linda and Jane need to jointly bring their concerns to their manager. The manager can do some investigation to see if Linda and Jane's perceptions are accurate. If the manager determines that Linda and Jane are indeed getting all the hard patients, he or she should take action.

Another thing the manager can do is provide a unit-wide mandatory in-service on mentoring and supporting new employees. New nurses could be assigned a designated mentor and champion who could help them with issues like the ones that Linda and Jane are facing. It might be necessary to draw up formal expectations regarding assignments for new nurses (for example, no more than one patient who is high acuity for the first 3 months). If the problem continues, a neutral party, such as a charge nurse on the previous shift, could be appointed to make the assignments, which are not subject to change by the nurses on the oncoming shift.

–Susan Johnson

After Jane and Linda share their concerns with the nurse manager, who can then monitor how work is being distributed. If their beliefs are legitimate, the manager needs to address the issue directly with those nurses who are taking advantage of Jane and Linda. It doesn't matter if you're new or experienced; what they're doing is taking advantage of their coworkers.

The thing that concerns me is that whoever made the assignments originally had a rationale for the way he or she did it; when other nurses change it, that's disrespectful to the scheduler. If the nurse manager made the assignments and assumed they were implemented as he or she created them, it will be a shock to discover they were altered.

If this practice continues, and the nurse manager is never made aware of what's going on, nothing will change. How the nurses approach him or her is critical, however. Maybe Jane and Linda could say, "I'm not sure if you're aware that after the assignments are made, they've been adjusted. If you're OK with this practice, that's fine, but we weren't sure if you knew this was happening."

The nurses who are making the changes need to be aware that if you're treating someone else unfairly, eventually the same thing will come back to you. It all goes back to what is fair.

–Kathy Curci

Reflection

How are patients assigned in your unit? Do unit politics make their way into the patient assignment? If so, what can you do to try to avoid this?

Do the nurses on your unit feel like patients are assigned in a fair way? Have you ever asked them? Do they have any ideas about how to make sure assignments are equitable?

Vignette 4.7: Favorites

The psych unit where Diane works often admits violent patients. Since there is a "no restraint" policy, nurses and technicians depend on each other to manage aggressive patients.

One day at work, Diane accidentally offends Julia, a co-worker, by interrupting her during a lunchtime conversation. Julia sees Diane's offense as one more in a series of rude behaviors and blows up at Diane. Diane realizes her mistake and quickly apologizes, to no avail.

Thereafter, Julia makes a point of helping every other nurse on the psych unit but ignoring Diane's requests. When a difficult patient is admitted and assigned to Diane, Julia tells Leon, a psych technician, to "help out," and walks away.

Expert Commentary: Vignette 4.7

Diane needs to bring her concerns to the manager. She can ask Leon and other witnesses to back her up. In this case, the manager might need to facilitate conversation between Diane and Julia (possibly with a neutral third party) to resolve the underlying issue that led to the problem. In addition, action plans can be developed for both Diane and Julia. The manager needs to make it clear to Julia that refusing to assist another coworker is not an option and might be grounds for disciplinary action. The manager or another party can also work with Diane on modifying her behavior so that she is no longer perceived as being rude.

–Susan Johnson

By not helping Diane in this situation, there is a real threat and danger of violence to her. If Julia doesn't help, Diane could be physically harmed. Something serious might happen; then, how would Julia feel?

When Julia was offended, Diane apologized right away, but it wasn't accepted, so she might wonder what she needs to do to be forgiven. Diane could ask Julia what would make her feel better, since an apology doesn't seem to have done the trick.

Regardless, it's wrong for Julia to leave her out on a limb and put her in harm's way because she's angry. A nurse might not always realize the consequences of his or her behavior, so it's advisable to think up-front about what you're risking—in this case, harm to a nurse from a patient.

–Kathy Curci

Reflection

Do you work in a unit where interpersonal conflict causes patient and staff safety issues? If yes, how have employees come to believe that this type of conflict is accecptable?

In health care, what factors lead a nurse to believe it is OK to put colleagues and/or patients at risk? As the nurse manager, what can you do to try to create a healthier working environment?

Vignette 4.8: The "In" Crowd

Every day at the visiting nurse association, Terri and Jess meet for lunch between patients. When other nurses are available at lunch time, Terri and Jess don't include them.

Sandy, a new nurse, helps pick up some cases from Terri's territory during a busy period. She asks Terri if they can meet for lunch and discuss the patients she will be taking over. "Oh, sorry, I'm meeting Jess for lunch," Terri answers.

Sandy doesn't think much of the decline until a few months later when she again has need of Terri's input on a patient. She asks about meeting over the lunch hour, and Terri again refuses. "You guys always go to lunch at the same time. How come I'm not invited?" Sandy asks.

"Jess and I have been friends forever, and we work really well together," Terri tells her. "You wouldn't understand anything we're talking about if you joined us." Sandy is hurt and confused but drops the idea of ever having lunch with Terri.

Expert Commentary: Vignette 4.8

There are two issues in this scenario: Sandy needs information from Terri regarding patients, and Jess and Terri's luncheon meetings exclude other staff. If the lunch meetings occur outside of work time, there is not much the manager can do about this. Employees are allowed to decide how they spend their off-duty time. There is no requirement that employees must be friends with each other outside of work, but they must be cordial at work. However, to facilitate friendships among all the staff, management might arrange some social events during work time, like a potluck, a pizza lunch, or an ice-cream social. To address the first issue, management needs to create formal mechanisms for staff to collaborate during work time. When nurses take over patients that another nurse has cared for, or if there is overlap in assignments, nurses must give report or have care conferences with each other. These meetings could be done in person, via phone, or via an electronic venue such as Skype.

–Susan Johnson

From a personal perspective, Sandy feels left out. But from a professional perspective, she needs information from Terri about a patient, and Terri needs to come up with an alternative way to provide it. It's on Terri to figure out how to address the need.

Do Terri and Jess have the kind of friendship where they can't include another person occasionally? They aren't being asked to share everything, but just one lunch. There may be some issues there in getting along with other colleagues in general. Sandy would at least understand the patient care things they are talking about, so it's an insult to suggest she wouldn't understand. Terri has put her down both personally and professionally.

It's good for all nurses to be sensitive to the fact that everyone wants to be included. If you extend yourself for this one person, you'll be glad you did if you need him or her to extend herself for you in the future. By including him or her, you open a door to an opportunity for this person to help you at some point.

–Kathy Curci

Reflection

Do some of your employees tend to spend off-work time, such as their lunch hour, with each other, to the exclusion of others? Do you think this is a bad thing? After all—they're just friends, right?

How might you—the nurse manager—handle a situation such as this one on your unit?

How does a nurse manager encourage a balance between professionalism and friendships among his or her staff?

Summary

Although nurses are adults, there can be a remarkable amount of high-school behavior on a unit. This might take the form of a campaign, in which a group of nurses gangs up on a coworker. Or it might be in the form of a drama queen, who deliberately stirs up trouble. Two-faced workers, who act pleasantly when in the company of management but terribly the rest of the time, are also a problem. Finally, the existence of cliques can have a negative effect on retention, not to mention lead to adverse symptoms among those left out.

Nurse managers must try to combat this behavior by encouraging staff to report it and ensuring those who do will not face retribution. Responding to this type of behavior can be really challenging, because it can feel murkey, unclear, or grey. Sometimes we might feel like something is wrong but can't quite put our finger on what. Often in these types of situations, careful and quiet reflection can lead to a better understanding of the problem. Nurse managers have to do their very best to make it clear that we are no longer in high school (thank goodness!), and that this type of behavior will not be tolerated. Specific strategies might include a unit-based council of role models or a zero-tolerance policy.

Activity

Research has shown that drama and cliques continue into the workplace, much as they did in high school. Challenge your staff members to take the opportunity to get to know their co-workers in a "Create a New Connection Day" where each nurse spends a few minutes talking with another nurse they don't know very well. You may even assign nurses to pairs where they must discuss an issue at work or just exchange a fun fact.

If possible, offer a motivator (such as a voucher for coffee or tea) to encourage these conversations.

Optional: If the opportunity presents itself, ask folks what fun thing they learned about their colleague.

5 | incivility

In recent years, many people have begun discussing the perception that interpersonal discourse has become increasingly uncivil—including in the workplace. Marlantes (2011) traces the roots of this discussion back to 1997, when the founder of the Public Conversations Project facilitated a retreat to discuss acrimony in the workplace. Now, so-called "civility coaches" offer their services to improve the emotional climate at your workplace, while career counselors help organizations create a culture of mutual respect. While the word *bullying* is often used interchangeably with the word *incivility*, we usually think of individuals who are aggressive, as opposed to environments that are intolerant. In any workplace, being uncivil involves a range of behaviors. Kirsten W. Schwehm (2006), university ombudsperson at Louisiana State University, suggests that incivility exists on a continuum from negative behavior (rude comments, spreading gossip or rumors, complaining) to verbal aggression (intimidating, discriminating, cursing, yelling) and then physical/sexual aggression. Depending on the intensity and frequency, these can add up to a toxic work environment.

Members of the Maryland Board of Nursing (BON) consider the issue of incivility so important that they created a Workplace Issues Subcommittee of the Commission on the Crisis in Nursing to look at the impact of "the culture of disrespect." They define civility as a behavior that is mutually respectful and leads to collaboration. A variety of individuals, such as nurses, physicians, and even patients and their families, can contribute to incivility, either directly or indirectly. Unfortunately, they believe that neither a nursing code of conduct nor a nursing code of ethics can address these behaviors fully.

Citing several studies that support the idea of civility and collaboration with positive patient outcomes, the BON encourages individual institutions to conduct a survey of all staff members on the quality of the emotional environment, as well as sponsoring discussion forums by experts. Existing policies on standards of conduct can be amended (with input from all employees) to include expectations of patients and families as well as health care team members. Finally, the BON suggested implementing a "civility board," which would have oversight of the organization and create the kind of infrastructure needed for reporting, reviewing, and responding to incivility. The BON notes that the orientation process and annual performance review are ideal venues for discussing civility and having staff sign a code-of-conduct policy (Maryland State Board of Nursing, 2005).

While gathering material for this book, we read a lot about workplaces with civility problems. Sometimes, it was a matter of one nurse "yelling" at another. In others, harsh comments were made in front of coworkers and/or patients. Communications that turned threatening or berating were also reported, along with physicians who verbally aggressed against nurses. (Note that almost all the aforementioned excellent suggestions from the BON related to nurses, not physicians.)

Another issue that fed into a negative environment in the workplace was organizational cynicism. Nurses who incessantly found fault with the management and/or organization and constantly suggested changes created a climate of dissatisfaction in the workplace. Judith Orloff (2005) describes people who leave you feeling "exhausted down to your very last molecule" as "energy vampires," a term that fits the feeling nurses described when confronted by coworkers who were bitter and organizationally cynical.

Yildirim (2009) found that nurse managers were often identified as a source of incivility, creating an environment that not only feels unsafe but affects a nurse's life both on and off the job. In a sample of 286 seasoned female nurses, 40% of those who were treated aggressively said that administrators were the bullies. Job motivation, energy level, and commitment to the job were significantly and negatively affected.

Russell (2012) offers these tips for increasing civility at the workplace:

- Identify positive role models who display the behaviors you seek. Administrators must lead the way in training themselves to act with civility.

- Take prompt action when you see incivility. Zero-tolerance policies are fine, but they're meaningless if they're not enforced.

- Encourage each employee to think about his or her level of civility. You might use a survey, a scenario, or a situation to prompt discussion on minimally acceptable workplace behaviors.

- Educate employees on anger and stress management techniques as well as communication. While some degree of conflict will always be present—perhaps even is healthy—you must understand when those emotional emails cross the line from encouragement to criticism.

- Weekly civility tips can reinforce desired behaviors.

- Pay attention to dress codes. There's some support for the idea that a sloppy appearance can result in diminishing professionalism.

- Be on time. If you're late, apologize.

- Ask for and be open to feedback on your performance. Encourage others to give you a civility report card every now and then.

We also encourage you to have a proactive plan in place so you can prevent crises. That way, when you see tension mounting or witness the potential for the deterioration of relationships, you can step in before an actual crisis occurs. This can be something entirely personal, or you can share it on a unit-wide level.

Commentator Beth Boynton notes the following:

In going from a toxic to healthy culture, key interventions include setting new norms, acknowledging and apologizing for past inappropriate behaviors, providing communication-skills training for all staff, creating opportunities for practicing and rewarding new behaviors, coaching individuals who may have a tougher time, and disciplining those who refuse to practice respectful behaviors. It is also crucial to have senior leadership support, no double standards, and a policy of "no innocent bystanders," making everyone accountable for respectful dynamics.

Ultimately, it is the nurse manager who will control the climate of an individual unit—often without much training in conflict management. Hopefully, working toward civility and away from conflict can be an approach that leads both patients and staff to communicate and interact respectfully in a way that makes everyone feel valued.

Vignettes, Commentaries, and Reflective Thinking

The remainder of this chapter presents vignettes about incivility, commentaries about the experiences represented in the vignettes, and opportunities to explore or reflect on the material.

Vignette 5.1: Too Loud

I sometimes work double shifts. On the 1600–2400 shift, there is a licensed practical nurse (LPN) who is well into her 60s. She has days where she is not as spunky and on top of things as other days. If it is a day where she needs more guidance, I try to be patient with her.

There is a registered nurse who becomes frustrated and has a short fuse with this LPN. I have witnessed on more than one occasion the RN degrading and yelling at the LPN, often in the hallway where the patients can overhear. Most times, the

LPN did not do anything to warrant the verbal abuse the RN bestowed upon her. The only outcome of the relational aggression as far as I can see is the LPN becomes more frustrated and less alert to tasks she is to do for patients.

One night, I was assigned to work with the LPN, and the RN was on the other team. There was an incident that involved the LPN with me and a volunteer. The RN tore down the hallway after the LPN and yelled at her. As soon as the RN returned to the nurse's station, I approached her. I pointed out to her that her behavior was inappropriate, and she had crossed the line and disrespected the LPN. The RN didn't want to hear about it, though, and she just walked away from me.

–Anonymous, BSN, RN-BC

Expert Commentary: Vignette 5.1

In this situation, it is right to be concerned about the RN's pattern of aggressive behavior toward the aging and possibly slower LPN. Anytime such behavior is tolerated, it is given silent permission to continue. The message goes to all stakeholders that such behavior is OK.

The most effective and direct way to address the incident would be for the concerned nurse to intervene while the hostile behavior is happening. In a clear and firm voice that everyone involved can hear, say "Stop yelling at her right now. Your behavior is inappropriate!" In this case, the offending RN, the LPN, and the volunteer all get the same message about the behavior. This type of intervention gets easier, although not necessarily easy, with practice and a supportive organizational culture. Later, take a quick, private moment with the LPN and volunteer to see if she is OK, and convey the message that no one deserves to be treated like that.

A private moment with the offending RN later in the shift would also be necessary. If the concerned nurse is a colleague, she might say, "I've been concerned about your yelling at the LPN for a while. It is harmful to all of us. If you continue, I am going to talk with the unit manager. If there is some way that I can be helpful, please let me know. If you have concerns about her performance, maybe you should talk with her or the unit manager. Do you understand what I am talking about?"

If the concerned nurse is a supervisor, a more authoritative tone and approach are warranted. She might say, "Yelling at the LPN is inappropriate. I am aware that I have tolerated your behavior for a while, and I was wrong to. I'm sorry if I have given you any ideas that abusive behavior is OK. It is not. Beginning now, I am going to call you on it and document it in your record. Do you know what I am talking about? Is there something that you need from me to behave more respectfully?"

Given the ongoing pattern of behavior witnessed by staff, patients, and volunteers, questions about the unit's organizational culture might occur to the nurse manager. This pattern of behavior includes multiple missed opportunities for the concerned nurse to give constructive feedback to the offending RN, LPN, and/or nurse manager and the LPN's unhealthy coping pattern of just walking away (a passive-aggressive action in its own way). In addition, there is the possible question of the LPN having performance issues. All these issues will have to be addressed.

–Beth Boynton

In this situation, the LPN who had been bullied by the RN is not spunky enough to stand up to the perpetrator. Although the LPN was warned by another nurse who witnessed the bullying, she still did not have the courage to stand up or even discuss the matter with the third person. I believe that by staying indifferent to her perpetrator, the LPN strengthens the RN's hand, which makes things even more miserable. In this case, the best thing is to inform the superiors and administration about the situation by a petition. That being said, the attitude of the administration is highly important to prevent these hostile behaviors. If administrators are determined enough to solve the LPN's problem, they will also prevent future bullying episodes.

–Dilek Yildirim

Reflection

Think about the "civility quotient" of your unit—how does it rate? What makes your staff more or less civil than others within the institution?

How far should a nurse manager go in intervening with interpersonal communication problems? Is it your job to make sure everyone on your unit gets along, or are there some times when employees need to figure things out for themselves?

Vignette 5.2: Rude Docs

Hector, a nurse on the rehabilitation unit, graduated from school the week before he started work. He is well received by his nurse coworkers, but the physicians give him a hard time. "You new nurses are all the same. No common sense!" fumes Dr. Monroe when Hector doesn't realize he is supposed to have his patient in bed when the physicians make rounds.

"If you had half a brain, you'd know that it's your job to make sure these patients take in enough calories to help them get through rehab!" says another doctor, Dr. Carter. "It's hard work to go through therapy all day."

Hector feels totally incompetent, even when the other nurses reassure him and try to run interference with the physicians.

Expert Commentary: Vignette 5.2

In this example, at least two doctors are known on the unit for berating new nurses. Sadly, many of us have experienced a transitional shock coming from a rigorous academic environment with a sense of accomplishment, excitement, and commitment to practice to this hostile and disrespectful "welcome" to the real-world nursing environment.

Stopping this disruptive behavior is crucial for collaboration, safe care, and for rewarding long-term careers. Ideally, the nurse manager would have spoken with these physicians individually prior to Hector's starting on the unit. A quick chat in private about the expectation of respectful behavior, sentinel event data related to poor communication, the cost of recruiting and retaining qualified staff, and an invitation to look at teaching opportunities as they arrive may be all that is needed. Because that didn't happen, the nurse manager will have to speak with Hector privately and explain that he or she is working on addressing this behavior with the physicians, that Hector should try not to take it personally, and that he or she would like to help Hector be assertive with these doctors the next time an incident occurs. They could use a scenario to role-play a response.

This would provide Hector with language and leadership support for the next time he is attacked by these doctors. Using a clear, firm voice and confident body language, Hector might say, "Dr. Monroe, your comments about all nurses lacking common sense are offensive. My goal is to work with you collaboratively for the safest and best care of our patients. I am happy to hear feedback on your preferences and concerns, and I expect you to treat me with respect. Can I count on you for this?" Or, "Dr. Carter, your insulting language is inappropriate. I agree that nutrition is an important factor of caring for our patients. There are many challenges associated with feeding patients, including their willingness to eat, the food, and the time and staff available to help. Let's schedule a meeting with the unit manager to discuss our concerns and address this issue."

Finally, the nurse manager should be aware that supportive staff by "running interference" may be contributing to an unhealthy alignment of us versus them with the physicians.

–Beth Boynton

While the claims of the physicians might be correct, the way they expressed them was inappropriate. Given the way the information was presented, the physician's rudeness could be considered bullying. Either way, I believe that Hector should talk to the physicians and tell them he was frustrated not by *what* they told him, but by *how* they told him.

–Dilek Yildirim

Reflection

How do physicians demonstrate respect for the skills of nurses in your organization and vice versa? Can you identify situations where "rude" interactions disrupted the work flow or caused emotional distress?

What is the difference between physicians who connect well with the nursing staff and those who do not? Think about specific behaviors they use and how you can help all team members be more explicit in supporting each other.

Vignette 5.3: Putdowns

Crystal, an LPN, is especially hostile toward young new nurses who are coming to work on the outpatient surgery unit. She has been at the unit for 20 years, and feels she is constantly put upon by fresh graduates who need to learn the policies and procedures. Lucy, one such new nurse, is a bit clumsy. During her first week in the unit, she trips and falls near a patient's bed. The next week, she bumps into Crystal when she's hurrying down the hallway with an armful of supplies.

When Lucy is trying to wheel a patient out of the unit in an oversized wheelchair and takes several tries to turn a corner, Crystal explodes. "How dumb are you?" she asks Lucy, pushing her out of the way and grabbing the handles of the wheelchair. "It's just not that hard to steer one of these around." The patient is shocked by the outburst, and Lucy dissolves into tears and flees to the bathroom.

Expert Commentary: Vignette 5.3

This is similar to the situation with Hector, except the disruptive behavior is coming from a seasoned LPN. In an ideal world, the nurse manager would have already addressed this behavior long before Lucy arrived but with new knowledge, must start when he or she can. In this case, the nurse manager could talk with Lucy privately to help her prepare to address inappropriate behavior. The nurse manager could also meet privately with

Crystal to set the tone for new expectations. An apology to the patient is also warranted. The nurse manager could suggest that Crystal apologize to the patient and Lucy together or separately.

The trick here is to recognize that such moments are filled with tension and awkwardness, yet are extremely therapeutic and powerful. Making the time for them, letting the tension settle for a few moments, and then moving on with clear, new expectations will help to minimize shame and maximize behavioral changes. It is also a management concern to be on the lookout for training needs of the new nurse and possibly job-match questions.

–Beth Boynton

I believe in most of the situations, Crystal has the right to react. But the reaction described here shows a lack of civility and a surplus of rudeness. I think Lucy should record the unfavorable events she has experienced in her new job and judge Crystal's attitude toward other nurses—especially fresh ones. She should also give some time to herself and Crystal to settle things down. But if Lucy is still getting the same rude reaction after a while—especially after she has found her footing and begun to act more responsibly—she should discuss the problem with Crystal and warn her about her impatient attitude with new nurses. Then, if Crystal's bad behavior persists, Lucy must go to the administration with her recorded events and ask them to warn Crystal about her rude attitude.

–Dilek Yildirim

Reflection

Do you believe rudeness between nurses of different rank or tenure is intentional? What are some ways to find out if insecurity or a sense of threat is the root cause of conflict and bullying, or more of a personality style?

Would the scenario with "Lucy" have evolved to the same intensity on your unit, or would you have intervened earlier? How have you handled the "Lucys" of nursing?

Vignette 5.4: Cynical Character

Gloria is a mature nurse and longtime employee on the pediatrics unit. She got her diploma at a 3-year school 30 years ago and has worked at the same hospital ever since. A series of mishaps have led Gloria to the edge of bankruptcy and divorce. Always a negative person, she has become downright bitter and speaks out at every opportunity.

"They don't care about nurses," she says when the hospital announces a temporary hiring freeze. "They just sit in their offices on their fat behinds and count dollars."

"She was a terrible nurse. We're better off without her," Gloria comments when Trinda, another longtime employee, transfers to the ED. "I can't imagine how she'll function with more work."

"This will be a terrible week, I can just tell," is Gloria's refrain on Monday mornings.

While some nurses have learned to ignore Gloria, some newer employees begin to feel stressed by her cynicism and pessimism.

Expert Commentary: Vignette 5.4

In this case, the nurse manager must address Gloria's negative behavior at work, despite awareness and concerns about her personal issues. Doing so can be tricky, but it's important to express concern about the latter while giving constructive feedback and possibly initiating disciplinary processes regarding the former. One way to do this would be for the nurse manager to set up a private meeting with Gloria to talk about some concerns she has. Offering to do this after work or giving the employee some choice, within reason, about when to meet would be a supportive gesture. In the meeting, the nurse manager might say something like this:

> *Gloria, I'm concerned about some negative and inappropriate comments I've heard you make and some of your colleagues have shared with me recently. One was about*

Trinda, and what a "terrible nurse" she was. Another was about the hiring freeze—something to the effect that "The hospital administration just sits in their offices on their fat behinds and count dollars." Do you know what I'm talking about? Can you understand why I am concerned?

Then pause. Let the feedback sink in. Gloria may have any number of reactions. She may get angry or teary, deny, apologize, or stay silent. After a moment, continue:

I expect you to stop these toxic comments, and I want you to consider this a verbal warning. Do you think you can put on a more positive attitude at work?

Pause again, before continuing:

I also want you to know that I am interested in your feedback or concerns you have about policies and procedures or even your colleagues' performance, and there is an appropriate time, place, and process for that. Are you willing to share your concerns in an appropriate way?

Once again, pause. Then say something like the following:

Lastly, I want you to know that I've heard through the grapevine that you are going through a rough patch at home. Is there some way I can help you? Have you considered using the employee assistance program or taking a few days off? You have a lot of valuable experience, and I'd like to find a way to keep you on the unit with a healthier attitude. Let's talk again in 2 or 3 weeks and see how things are going.

Culture change is hard work and requires trust, complex human behaviors and relationships, and a long-term commitment. In the long run, units that undergo this type of culture change will be safer, staff morale will be better, patient and family experiences will be optimal, and care will be more cost-effective.

–Beth Boynton

I think Gloria is not a person that others would be happy to work with. Her cynical and pessimistic character influences everyone in the work environment and makes the atmosphere unfavorable to fruitful work. I strongly believe that anyone who influences the work environment in this way, affecting others' performance, should not be on the team. Before taking serious steps, however, the nurse manager has to talk to Gloria about her problems and her attitude toward her superiors and colleagues. I would warn her about the unfavorable effects of her attitude on the other staff. If Gloria insists on continuing with her behavior, I would ask her to leave. I strongly believe in the importance of a harmonious work environment. It is important not only for the staff's health, but also for the patients' safety.

–Dilek Yildirim

Reflection

Does negativity on your unit come from interpersonal conflicts or environmental influences? That is, does negativity skyrocket when nurses are busier than usual or around the holidays, or do a few bad apples create an ongoing toxic environment?

Do you as a nurse manager role model a positive attitude? When you're upset with a particular situation or person, what would your staff say about the way you respond?

Summary

As the nurse manager, you create a climate that impacts those who work for and with you. By recognizing that both employees and those they serve can be a source of rudeness and incivility, having a response plan in place will help you avoid having to scramble when an event occurs.

Promoting good relationships among all members of your team is also part of the nurse manager's job. Being a combination of cheerleader and coach, as well as demonstrating loyalty and commitment to those you supervise, will build a foundation of positive relationships throughout.

Activity

Poll your staff about key behaviors that reflect civility. Ask them to write down two or three important things that they believe demonstrate a sense of civility between coworkers. You can do this anonymously so people will feel comfortable being honest. Summarize the responses and explore the idea of a "civility behavior contract" between coworkers, and accountability checks for incivility. You can do the same with expectations for civility toward and from patients and family members or other visitors.

part II relationship riff

6 | competition and credit

Some of the issues discussed in this chapter may seem like small ones. As commentator Victoria Schirm puts it, "These examples address issues that are frequently found on nursing units, and at first glance seem rather trivial amid the life and death situations that are encountered today in many acute care hospitals." Nevertheless, Schirm continues, "each situation, if avoided or ignored, has potential for adverse consequences for the nursing workforce and patient care."

It's human nature to be proud of one's own work. When we work hard on a product, we want our name attached to it so our colleagues and managers know that we worked hard and we delivered. In short, we all want credit where credit is due.

This perspective, however, must be balanced against a teamwork philosophy, in which the primary goal is the health and well-being of the team, not the individual. When you think about things from the perspective of the team, you may find the picture shifting a bit. This is not to say that individuals should not receive recognition for their accomplishments. Ideally, individuals *should* receive recognition, but often, innovations and ideas become bigger than the individual who conceived them, as the team works to take their work to the next level. Think of it this way: When a soccer player scores a goal, we acknowledge and reward that player's performance, but we also recognize that the goal could not have been scored without the support of the other players on the field.

Competition can exist not only in the day-to-day work of nurses, but also within the salary and promotion structure. As an example, consider a second-career nurse who was recently hired to a new position in a new institution. One piece of information she wanted to know was how her salary and benefits package compared to other people who were recently hired into similar positions. This information would give her insight into how she rated in comparison to her peers, as well as an idea of her "worth" to the institution.

Still, discovering that your peers make more money than you do can lead to resentment and confusion. Why are you being compensated less for doing essentially the same job? Competition over salary and promotions can be an important source of conflict in the current economy, even in unionized environments.

Another area of rivalry is over upward mobility within the organization. The idea that nursing could be a career path is a relatively new one, but given clinical ladders and a variety of graduate programs that connect work product to merits, it's now realistic to think about nursing in this way.

One potential barrier to teamwork is the fact that the nursing workforce remains predominantly female. This results in women competing with other women for jobs, advancement, and credit. Nan Mooney (2005), author of *I Can't Believe She Did That! Why Women Betray Other Women at Work*, noted, "It's been such a taboo subject. To say women have problems with each other is seen as antiwoman, but it's not. Why is it so hard to work with other women? Why are we so nasty to each other?" If this sentiment strikes you as antiwomen, then you're in good company—some commentators are critical of Mooney's work for just this reason. Additionally, research from Catalyst shows that senior female executives consistently point to gender-based stereotyping as a major barrier to their advancement (Armour, 2005).

Three main theories may help explain the friction between women in the workplace:

- **Getting along:** Many women are socialized to be nice to others, to be ladylike, not to fight, and to compromise. As a result, women in the workforce tend to compete while simultaneously acting like they're *not* competing. This can lead to passive-aggressive behaviors and even backstabbing.

- **Communication:** Many women form interpersonal relationships by sharing intimate details of their lives. This can come back to haunt them, however. As discussed in Chapter 4, "Cliques, Campaigns, and High-School Drama," nurses—like all people—engage in gossip frequently.

- **Scarcity:** There aren't a whole lot of top-notch positions for women.

It seems that a foundational question that we must ask—one that has not yet been definitively answered—is, in the workplace, are women sometimes their own worst enemies (Armour, 2005)? Psychologist Vivian Diller (2012) argues:

> *More often than not, women would do better if they joined together to share concerns—be it professional or personal—rather than battle each other about them. Older women can mentor younger ones, teach them from experience how to balance work, relationships, and motherhood. Younger women have a lot to learn from their older colleagues, and gain more from being supportive of them knowing that they too will be there someday.*

One of the ways competition and rivalry manifest in the nursing workplace is through the taking of another nurse's supplies or resources. We read many bitter complaints about coworkers who hoard linens or other scarce items, monopolize machinery, and walk away with a careful collection of supplies needed for a procedure. Another manifestation occurs on the relationship level. Nurses who aggressively jockey for status or promotion are criticized, as are units that compete on a macro (institutional) level for rewards and recognition.

Vignettes, Commentaries, and Reflective Thinking

The remainder of this chapter presents vignettes about competition and credit, commentaries about the experiences represented in the vignettes, and opportunities to explore or reflect on the material.

Vignette 6.1: Taking Credit

Jen develops a new discharge teaching plan for patients with newly diagnosed diabetes as part of her graduate research course. After conducting a review of the literature, she creates learning objectives and a curriculum that any nurse can use to prepare patients for self-care.

She leaves a copy of the completed paper with her nurse manager. "I'd like your thoughts on this as a possible tool for us to use," she says on the sticky note attached to the front of her paper. When Selma, her nurse manager, doesn't reply, Jen asks some of the other nurses on the medical floor where she works part time if they know anything about the program she proposed.

"You mean the new discharge teaching plan?" Flora responds. "Selma presented that to us at our last staff meeting and said management is all in favor of using it. I thought she developed it!"

Jen confronts Selma about distributing the teaching plan without giving her credit. Selma is amused. "Jen, we're a team here," Selma says. "We all work together, and no one person gets special credit."

Expert Commentary: Vignette 6.1

The irony of this situation with Jen and Selma is the apparent lack of teamwork on both sides. The lack of an in-person conversation between them regarding use of the teaching tool contributed to a failure in collaboration. On the one hand, Selma appears to have taken advantage of Jen's action of leaving the teaching tool with only a sticky note. Without direction from Jen, Selma seemingly used the opportunity to implement a program that she recognized as good for the unit. Of course, such an action might occur in a manager's hectic schedule of executing the day-to-day operations of a busy nursing unit, but this would have the inadvertent consequence of failing to promote team partnerships.

At the same time, Jen followed up not with Selma, but with other nurses with whom she works. This misdirected communication falls short of the mark to communicate with the individual who has the information about the situation. Another issue that can be raised is why Jen left it so open regarding the teaching plan, with only a sticky note requesting a response. Was Jen unsure of the value of her work and how it would be received? If it was rejected or otherwise not used, would Jen have responded differently? Is Selma, the nurse manager, unapproachable, or not readily available to nursing staff? Answers to these questions may provide insight into how teamwork is valued on the unit.

–Victoria Schirm

Because Selma is Jen's nurse manager, this situation is especially delicate. Certainly, nurse managers are often in a position of heading up projects that involve employees, but guidelines need to be clearly established ahead of time.

For example, Selma may have already recognized the need for this kind of teaching program and just hadn't gotten around to planning a committee or asking for volunteers to work on creating it. Perhaps she even introduced the tool as Jen's creation or modified it to conform to administrative guidelines for performance. If this is the case, she should promptly share those details with Jen. It could even be that Jen heard Selma talking about the need for a better teaching plan, and decided to act on it. Clearer communication on both sides might dispel misunderstandings that led to this conflict.

That being said, Jen has devoted a lot of work to the project, and the work that currently exists rightfully belongs to her. She has every reason to go to Selma's manager and explain the situation. At a minimum, her efforts deserve recognition and a request for her permission to use it.

Selma's comment about being a "team" makes me wonder if other issues haven't cropped up on her unit. When one person does most or all of the work on a given day or for a given project, it's a failure of the team concept. It might be worth a discussion at the next staff meeting so all nurses are clear on what her expectations are. As a nurse manager, having all the nurses who work with you recognized for their work is a better reflection of your effectiveness than any individual glory.

–Cheryl Dellasega

Reflection

When is it appropriate for you or another nurse manager to take credit for innovations that emerge from your unit?

How transparent should a nurse manager be to his/her staff? Do you need to justify your evaluations and recommendations of staff, even when they comply with the organization's policy?

If one of your staff confronted you about selecting one nurse to represent the unit at a local conference, how would you respond?

Vignette 6.2: Thief

The nurses at Hope Hospital have a love-hate relationship with the student nurses who are assigned to shifts throughout the hospital. While they appreciate the extra help, they become irritated at having to take time to help students learn the ropes.

Maura, who works on a medical floor, is famous for "hiding" laundry from the students so they are unable to change beds or provide care. When they come to her for help, she pretends not to know where the linens are and won't tell the students how to obtain more. Later, when the instructor comes on the floor, Maura makes sure to tell her the students are providing sloppy care. She says, "They didn't bother to change bed linens or give their patients a towel and washcloth."

Expert Commentary: Vignette 6.2

Necessary interactions between students and experienced nurses frequently produce angst. The troublesome attitudes and feelings that arise on the part of nursing staff may stem from past experiences with students or from recollections of the nurse's own student days. Mistaken notions may exist that the intimidation of others makes oneself look or feel good, or such actions are attempts to create self-worth or importance.

This scenario suggests that at Hope Hospital, an apparent negative culture exists between nurses who feel obligated to contribute to the education of nursing students, yet are resentful when it is time to participate. The undermining and sabotaging are disruptive not only to the learning experience, but also to quality patient care and safety.

In this situation, the nurse manager needs to effectively set the direction for accountability among all involved. As the leader for the unit, the nurse manager is in a position to promote dialogue among nursing staff, nursing faculty, and students. A first step in the process may be an examination of the overall unit culture of reward and recognition. For example, are staff nurses themselves receiving limited praise, encouragement, or support? What daily vexations and disappointments may be contributing to the contentious culture with students?

Approaches to the resolution of existing conflicts entail nurse managers fully understanding their intended outcome. Creating success for one side or the other frequently continues the status quo. Focus needs to be on what is beneficial for the team. One component of the process is to ensure that leaders are respectful—and through that respect create awareness that management and staff care about the same things. A second component is to clarify and avoid incorrectly identifying or assuming knowledge of intentions. Acknowledge that all participants' contributions are important to the team. A third element is to keep to the facts and avoid beliefs, opinions, and impressions that create emotional reactions. Not to be overlooked in resolving issues is following up.

This case provides an example of applying these steps. It is apparent that avoidance of confronting the discontent is not working but is permitting continuation of the status quo. The nurse manager has an opportunity to take the lead in focusing on how the disparate groups can become part of a team. A meeting of nursing staff and nursing faculty could be a first step, with focus given to creating awareness that both groups want to foster good experiences for nursing students.

–Victoria Schirm

The nursing instructor is, in effect, a manager of students in the clinical area. By observing closely to make sure the work is being done correctly by those in training, staff nurses won't need to report problems.

Of course, there are times when an instructor may not be on the scene as the Mauras of the world fail to support new learners. In that case, the educator needs to immediately check with the students to get their input. Once the cause of this conflict is determined, the next step is for the instructor to go to the nurse manager, who, most likely, has already received similar complaints about Maura.

It is the nurse manager's job to help his or her staff recognize the contributions that nursing students can make to a clinical unit. If there is an attitude of hostility toward students, that site might not be the best place for new learners. The nurse manager is responsible for ensuring that his or her staff is a source of support, not stress, for students.

Written guidelines can be helpful here. A document that spells out the expectations of students as well as staff can guide both groups ahead of time. This kind of policy or procedure could be developed jointly by the nurse educator and the nurse manager. A thorough orientation to the unit for students and introductions to the nurses they will be working with can also help.

–Cheryl Dellasega

Reflection

What do nurses ethically "owe" to those who are coming up in the profession? Should practicing nurses be expected to educate students in addition to their other responsibilities? If so, should they receive special training?

How well do you work with nurse educators and other visitors to your unit? Is there a policy about how these relationships should play out during work hours?

Vignette 6.3: The Biggest Contest

Several young nurses are eagerly anticipating the July letter that announces their yearly salary increase. Although no one actually shares their salary, each nurse wonders what the other makes.

Anita, an RN who recently finished her BSN, announces that her nurse manager has promised to be "generous" given the additional educational efforts she has made. The other nurses on Anita's floor, however, feel she is lazy and doesn't provide good care to critically ill elderly patients.

Resentment against Anita builds. The other nurses complain among themselves about the raises they didn't get—at her expense. Soon, morale is low and the staff refuses to work with Anita, who continues to brag about her many accomplishments in and out of school.

Expert Commentary: Vignette 6.3

The resentment toward Anita is unfortunate, as is the apparent lack of nurse-manager involvement in bettering the situation. The nurse manager is in the position to convey the organization's fundamental nondiscriminatory principles and procedures regarding salary and evaluations. Staff's disgruntled and complaining behavior among themselves, without communication and clarification with the nurse manager, intensifies the state of affairs. Improving the situation requires transparency on the part of the nurse manager and communicating that objective criteria are used for salary adjustments and performance evaluations. Anita's behavior needs to be handled rather than allowing the continued complaining among staff. The resulting lack of teamwork and diminished morale creates an untenable situation, where nurse dissatisfaction has the potential to affect patient care, satisfaction, and safety.

–Victoria Schirm

This situation is obviously unique to nonunion or non-collective-bargaining worksites. If there are mandated raises and standards for job performance, the discussion of salaries and promotions that results in jealousy, resentment, and hurt probably will not be an issue. (This is not a plug for unions, however!)

Nonetheless, transparency in all aspects of oversight should be a guiding principle for nurse managers. Hiring, evaluation, and termination procedures should be documented and shared freely with employees. There should be consistency on the part of the nurse manager, so no single nurse feels as if he or she is treated differently or unfairly.

A bit of competition can be a good thing, though. Periodically recognizing nurses for an exemplary job or a special contribution can show that you *do* value the employee who goes above and beyond the minimal expectations. A public acknowledgement of Anita and everyone who pursues additional education would be helpful. A firm statement about procedures for evaluating employees and determining annual raises could also help address any other undercurrents of tension.

–Cheryl Dellasega

Reflection

What is "confidential" information regarding salary and status? Is it appropriate for a nurse manager to tell her staff to, in essence, "mind their own business," or does he/she have an obligation to share the rationale behind these decisions?

How transparent are your own interactions with your peers? Do nurse managers at your institution share information about their salaries and benefits? Should they?

Vignette 6.4: Overdrive

Trudy works in the ICU but wants to "move up" to a management position. She is taking graduate courses toward her MSN but also seeks out opportunities to position herself as a leader at the worksite.

After one harrowing afternoon with two codes and many unstable patients, the nurse manager, Bev, makes a point of telling all the ICU nurses that she appreciates their efforts and perseverance. "We couldn't do this kind of work if we weren't a team," she summarizes as the shift ends.

Bev and most of the day nurses leave, but Trudy stays behind. She sees Norma, the nursing supervisor for the evening shift, approaching the ICU on rounds.

"I hear it was chaotic here today," Norma says.

"Yes, it was," Trudy replies. "I worked really long and hard and wanted to stay and make sure all my charting was current. I volunteered to take an extra patient and pretty much ran the unit while the others were tied up with the codes."

Norma smiles and gives Trudy a "thumbs up." The next day, Dottie, the day supervisor for the ICU, sees Bev in the hallway. "You know, we've got our eye on Trudy. She's a really good nurse and so hardworking. Norma got another glowing report on her last night."

Bev pauses, not certain what to say. She agrees that Trudy is a good nurse and hard worker, but feels she is not the best nurse in the ICU. Dottie's comment concerns her, because she's seen Trudy take full credit for teamwork in the past.

Expert Commentary: Vignette 6.4

Trudy's individual determination to excel appears to be at the expense of the overall recognition for teamwork that Bev wants to promote on the unit. The conversation related to the praise and credit given to Trudy leaves Bev with the impression that the unit's successful teamwork is being attributed to the work of one individual. In her experience, Bev recognizes that this instance is similar to past behavior on the part of Trudy. Such an understanding can be a prompt for Bev to have a conversation with Trudy to seek clarification on the details conveyed about the "hectic day." The conversation between Norma and Trudy does not necessarily reflect an overstatement of taking undue credit. Bev needs to discuss her views of the current situation with Trudy, and share her beliefs about similar situations that have occurred in the past.

Nurse managers need to model behavior to overcome the conflicts. This skill set includes asking clarifying questions, listening attentively, allowing all to speak, giving the benefit of the doubt. Analyzing the information affords the opportunity for resolutions that promote teamwork. The ability to execute these elements—many of which are part of a nursing assessment—requires practice.

–Victoria Schirm

Everyone seems to encounter a Trudy sometime in life—a person whose ambition overwhelms and irritates his or her coworkers. As a nurse manager, the balance between supporting staff members who are more "self-promoting" in their efforts and curtailing behavior that detracts from teamwork can be challenging.

Bev might deal with the situation by having a follow-up conversation with both Norma and Dottie to emphasize that Trudy *is* doing a good job—as are other nurses on the unit. A reiteration of the events of the day of the double codes could illustrate how everyone worked together, *including* Trudy, but not *especially* Trudy.

Being fortunate to have a group of nurses who can pull together during difficult times is a reflection of the manager's ability to inspire them and reinforce cohesion. Taking other opportunities to emphasize the value of the team when Trudy is present is important—but there could be an offer to provide her, and anyone else interested, with concrete chances to do some extra work assignments that would showcase her/their talents and special interests.

–Cheryl Dellasega

Reflection

How can nurse managers obtain information about what happens on their units when they aren't physically present? How do you decide who is trustworthy, and who is not?

What can a nurse manager do to balance ambition in her staff? What can you do to encourage nurses to set goals and achieve them, continuously improve, but avoid being obnoxious as they do so?

Summary

Nurse managers want the very best from their staff, which means balancing the right amount of professional challenge with an individual employee's abilities. Deciding how and when to intervene in situations that challenge those who work for you requires wisdom, tact, and careful timing.

At the same time, you need to feel like you are leading, not prodding or curtailing, your staff. Sometimes your job might feel more like soothing a group of tired preschoolers than facilitating the professional development of nurses, but the best leaders inspire by example rather than punishing or ignoring bad behavior.

Ultimately, a sense of teamwork will help everyone to function at the top of their game. Finding the "glue" of quality patient care that can bind together students, physicians, and nurses is a strategic move that makes a nurse manager an effective leader.

Activity

The goal here is to build a sense of teamwork. One way to do this is to create teams of nurses and have friendly competition for a small reward. Here are some ideas:

- Divide the unit into two teams and give everybody a pedometer. See which team covers the most mileage—on and off the job—in 1 week.

(continues)

(continued)

- Work with another unit manager to collect canned goods for a worthy cause. Make it clear that each unit is a team, and they should be in it to win it. See who can collect the most cans.

- Adopt a worthy cause, and figure out ways your unit can work together to raise funds or promote health.

7 | personal issues and downtime behavior

Nurses are great at taking care of others, but not so good at taking care of themselves. Gessler and Ferron state, "The most important thing nurses can do for themselves, their patients, and the people they love is to make self care a priority" (2012). He encourages empowerment of nurses through the following:

- Clear and available guidelines for reporting violations in the workplace with a follow-up mechanism

- An ombudsperson

- Effective communication skills

- Mentoring programs for experienced nurses to help newbies

- A wellness committee

On the organizational level, help with managing work stress can be offered through employee assistance program (EAP) efforts that focus on wellness, coaching, assertiveness training, availability of counseling, and peer coaching.

It behooves the nurse manager to constantly monitor the status of the unit he or she is in charge of, assessing the emotional climate and relationships between coworkers. Stress management for both oneself and others is also an important tool that can quickly address day-to-day events that accumulate and overwhelm. During times of crisis or tension, it is all too easy for the person in charge to get swept up in the emotion of the moment. Being aware of your own strengths and weaknesses is an important management strategy.

In 2009, the Joint Commission created a standard that was intended to curb bullying and other bad behaviors in the health care workplace. It encouraged education of employees about professional behavior, leadership training, and providing a mechanism for reporting aggressive behavior (Lally, 2009). However, nurses have noted that when accreditors such as Magnet reviewers are visiting, input from individual nurses is solicited in a public way. Bringing up personal issues that sully the workplace or speaking negatively about coworkers can seem inappropriate in this venue, and fear of retribution often prevents honest disclosures that might be more forthcoming in private venues.

The boundary between personal and professional is increasingly blurred during off-duty hours as nurses take to blogs to express frustrations or celebrate accomplishments. Using one's real name and sharing information that would permit the reader to identify a specific hospital and/or patient are problematic, opening the author to potential stalkers or harassment.

Revealing patient information can also violate HIPAA laws regulating privacy. A nurse may think it is OK to post a picture or video from work without being aware that it could contain patient identifiers in the form of images or information associated with a particular hospital. Even a signature or chart information might be inadvertently included in an image or the text of a blog.

The National Council of State Boards of Nursing (NCSBN) issued a white-paper guideline on social media that describes the use of social media by nurses (NCSBN, 2011). It discusses the difference between confidentiality and privacy. Confidential information is shared during the clinical relationship but may not be shared beyond the treatment team under most circumstances. Privacy, on the other hand, is the patient's right to be treated with dignity and respect through a relationship of trust. NCSBN also describes the possible consequences of misuse of social media. Although each case would be decided by the state board of nursing, there could be disciplinary action in the form of a reprimand or sanction, fine, and even loss of licensure.

Students and other job seekers need to be wary of what they post on public forums. It's reasonable for employers to check out would-be employees online and make judgments about their compatibility with a particular institution or organization. Once employed, it still behooves an individual nurse to be cautious about what he or she posts, particularly at work, because the employer may screen outgoing emails and posts with software designed for that purpose.

Legal action has been taken when a nurse used social media during work time. In *Chapman v. Unemployment Compensation Board of PA* ("Cell Phones," 2011), an RN was fired from her position in a nursing home because she used her personal phone to post information about a coworker on Facebook. The timestamp on her Facebook post revealed it was posted at work. Because her employer had a policy against using personal cell phones at work, as well as the stated right to immediately terminate anyone who violated this rule, the court ruled it was not a violation of privacy to check her Facebook page. They ruled in favor of the employer, especially when the nurse admitted to accessing the Internet and posting at the same time she was giving out medications.

Fortunately, this employer had well-articulated policies that spelled out the specifics of cell-phone use in the workplace. The larger organization will most likely establish these institution-wide guidelines, but nurse managers can provide input on his or her reasonable expectations. It goes without saying that he or she needs to model the desired behaviors both on the job and off.

NCSBN (2011) suggests these guidelines when creating policy:

- Patient safety comes first.
- Nurses must act ethically and legally.
- No patient images or information may be shared.
- Be aware of the institutional and patient reputation when sharing information.

- No photographs should be taken at the workplace on employee cell phones.

- Consider professional behavior when communicating electronically with patients or former patients.

- Be prompt in reporting any violations.

- Do not make disparaging comments about employers or coworkers.

At the same time, cell phones and social media can be of great help. Many nurses use cell phones in particular as drug guides or language translators. Nurses can use social media as an informal source of support, connecting with colleagues around the world. While there may be policies related to cell-phone use, the reality is often very similar to schools, where students are told phones are banned but everyone has them. Ignoring the reality of employees using cell phones and social media is not an option.

Another aspect to consider with regard to nurses' personal lives is when nurses experience problems at home that spill over into their work lives. Spousal unemployment, divorce, caregiving, emotional problems with family, and an array of other situations can make a nurse's on-the-job performance subpar. The nurse manager is often put in a position of needing to balance being supportive with following human-resources policies and procedures. Being aware of options for leave and other alternatives can help in these situations.

Vignettes, Commentaries, and Reflective Thinking

The remainder of this chapter presents vignettes about personal issues and downtime behavior, commentaries about the experiences represented in the vignettes, and opportunities to explore or reflect on the material.

Vignette 7.1: Private Talk

Megan, a new nurse who is young and inexperienced, often uses her downtime to make personal calls on her cell phone. When Rick, her nurse manager, sees her in the hallway laughing and spending time in conversation with a friend on the phone, he calls her into his office.

"Unless it's an emergency, we don't encourage use of personal cell phones here, Megan. It doesn't look professional to patients and visitors or other staff."

"But I didn't have any work to do," Megan counters. "It was a slow day, and no one but you saw me on my phone."

Rick relents and tells her she still needs to be more discreet. The next time he makes rounds, he finds her in the nurses' lounge, talking on her phone. It's not hard to figure out that the call is personal.

Expert Commentary: Vignette 7.1

At first glance, this simply seems like a generational issue. Millennial/Generation Y nurses, who are broadly defined as those born in the 1980s and 1990s, are tech-savvy, with a cell phone practically surgically attached. It is not uncommon to see a table of millennials in a restaurant, all on their cell phones, texting each other and other friends who are not with them, rather than having a face-to-face conversation with each other. During a nursing class, I often look around the large lecture hall and see students busily texting each other on their cell phones. When I've spoken to students about cell-phone use during class, I am told that they are able to pay attention to the class while using their cell phones. One student became quite irate when I asked her to stop using her phone. Acceptable social morals have shifted with such lightning speed that baby boomers cannot keep up with the new rules. When these Generation Y/ millenial students graduate, they naturally take these new rules to their workplace.

The young nurse in this vignette was only doing what she has always done. She is so accustomed to using her cell phone to stay socially connected at all times that it is likely that she sees nothing wrong or unusual with her behavior. She does not see that once one enters the workplace, the rules change. In all but the most informal work settings, personal telephone conversations are limited to matters that cannot wait until the end of the work day, and it is expected that such conversations be kept very short.

As a manager, I would first check the agency policy to be certain I was not enforcing a policy contrary to what is already in place. Assuming there was no written policy related to cellphone use, I would have a staff meeting to allow all personnel an opportunity to voice their opinion. Hopefully, the group could come to a consensus and understand that personal calls while on duty are inappropriate.

The main points that should be made at such a meeting are as follows:

- A hospital is a workplace like any other. It is not a place for personal business.

- The nature of patient care is such that one's work is never done. If all tasks are completed, this presents a perfect time for the nurse to spend a few minutes talking to a patient who is alone and frightened, has no visitors, is facing a difficult diagnosis, or just needs additional attention.

- Personal calls should be reserved for urgent matters, should take place on the hospital desk phone, and should be limited to 3 to 5 minutes.

- Calls on one's personal cell phone should take place off the clinical unit during break or lunch time.

Once everyone knows the policy, it is then reasonable to expect that all staff members adhere to it. Any further use of cell phones while on duty will be dealt with in the same way as any other violation of policy.

–Shellie Simons

Like Rick, I would discuss with Megan what happened when she was having the personal conversation in the public workplace and how it looked to the patients and families who saw her. Regarding the second incident, it is important to know whether Megan was on her break when she was in the lounge. If she was not on a break and others needed her assistance, that could be the topic of the conversation. If she *was* on her break, I would ask what the harm is with her taking a personal call in the breakroom. If cell phones are not prohibited in the lounge for a reason, is it a problem for them to be used there? While we need to maintain boundaries and create a professional workplace, we must remind ourselves how important connectivity has become to our staff, regardless of age. Appropriate location of cell-phone use could be the topic of focus. I would encourage Rick to review the hospital policy on cell-phone use in the health care setting. I also would encourage him to discuss the use of cell phones with his peers to determine whether it is also a problem on their units. This would provide the opportunity to discuss as a leadership group what they believe is the right thing to do about the use of technology in the workplace. Staff can also provide input and participate in the decisions regarding their work environment.

The use of technology in the workplace has become increasingly important to all of us who work in health care. We are challenged to learn new technology to better care for our patients and their families. We also have become more connected in our personal lives. We must consistently look at how we can balance the need to be connected with our professional obligation to our patients, families, and coworkers.

In the past, cell phones and other wireless technology affected many of the devices used in an acute-care setting, such as ventilators, monitors, etc. That is not necessarily the case any longer. Most health care technology is not affected by our wireless devices. Our practices often need to be reevaluated when we introduce new equipment to determine whether we need to change our processes and procedures.

As technology advances, we also need to consider the advantages to having staff carry their smart devices in the workplace. Technology has made accessing important information even more easy and reliable by "creating an app for that." Nurses may now access drug dosing, check medication interactions, etc., all with their phones. This advancement in technology has become and will continue to be a tool to enhance patient safety.

The balance of creating a healthy work environment is a difficult situation. We need to think about what is important to our staff and weigh that with the right thing to do in our health care environment. We have often taken a black-and-white stance on things and need to look at what the decision is for those affected. As nurse leaders, we must provide guidance and consistency and ask the appropriate questions to create an environment in which people want to work, while maintaining a professional standard in our work unit.

–Patti Hart

Reflection

How can nurses—especially younger ones—balance the need to use technology as part of their job with their desire to use technology to communicate socially? Do you handle personal calls on the cell phone in the same way you handled those on a landline?

If your hospital expects nurses to communicate with other team members via cell phone, how do you avoid becoming the cyber police, monitoring every call that is made during the workday? How do you strike the balance between supporting technology while also opposing bad technology behavior?

Vignette 7.2: Family Crisis

Lori's elderly mother has been acutely ill with pancreatic cancer, which has taken a toll on Lori, the family "nurse." Many days, Lori comes to work on the rehabilitation floor with tired eyes and obvious fatigue. One morning, she leaves the side rail of an elderly patient's bed down, and the man falls out of the bed.

Lori's nurse manager, Bree, suggests that Lori consider taking family medical leave to provide care for her mother, but Lori says that's impossible. "We need every extra penny we can find to drive my mother to and from the city for chemo," she protests. "My parents are retired and on a fixed income. They were barely scraping by before this."

Bree is worried that because Lori is so distracted and tired, her work is suffering. Bree takes Lori aside and expresses this concern. Lori says she understands and will do her best, but Bree is still worried that Lori might make a serious mistake that could result in poor patient care or, worse, litigation.

Expert Commentary: Vignette 7.2

In this scenario, it is not stated whether Lori is a longtime employee with outstanding skills, a nurse with low energy and passable skills, or a new employee barely through the probationary period. These specifics would provide some guidance as to how the manager might proceed.

In any case, a nurse who is tired or distracted and cannot leave personal problems at home is a danger to his or her patients. Recently, I was with a student as she was preparing to administer medications, and she accidentally retrieved the wrong dose of heparin. After correcting the error, I sat with the student to discuss the incident privately. She told me that a beloved relative was gravely ill, and she couldn't stop worrying about her relative. I explained to her that because she was so distracted, she should have stayed home and taken care of her personal business. She argued that she would then have missed a clinical and did not want to make it up. She thought it best to "come and try to do her best."

Later that day, we talked about this with the entire group. I explained to the group that nursing was not like some other jobs, where if you make an error because you're distracted, it can easily be fixed without serious consequence. The group agreed that when a nurse makes an error, a patient could be seriously injured or worse. It is the professional responsibility of all nurses to be focused and alert when reporting for duty. If, for whatever reason, he or she is not, the nurse needs to be responsible and stay home.

That said, a manager needs to evaluate the strengths of the staff member in question to know how to best act in this scenario. Assuming this nurse has a good work history and has proven to be a valuable asset to the unit, the manager would be inclined to do whatever is possible to assist her through this difficult period without compromising patient safety.

The manager could meet with Lori and tell her that she will make reasonable accommodations, but that it is Lori's professional responsibility to come to work alert and focused. Lori can also be referred to employee assistance. Employee assistance is set up to help employees through difficult situations and may be able to refer this employee to resources that can aid her with her difficult home situation.

The manager can also offer a flexible schedule with temporarily reduced hours. Perhaps clustering Lori's scheduled hours over 2 or 3 days will give her the time needed at home. Some work settings allow employees to donate a day of earned time to another employee going through difficult times. If the agency permits, this could be suggested to other staff members. If Lori has a history on this unit, it is likely her coworkers would be eager to assist her in this way.

In any case, nursing is a caring profession, and it is essential that we demonstrate a caring attitude when one of our own is facing a difficult situation. By showing compassion and a sincere attempt to offer assistance, the manager is modeling the behavior that she wants all her staff to exhibit toward each other and their patients.

Hopefully, Lori will be able to figure out how to better handle the stress she is facing at home while continuing to work. In the end, though, if none of these solutions work, and Lori continues to be exhausted and distracted, the manager has no choice but to insist that Lori take a family medical leave until the crisis has passed. Ultimately, the manager must protect the patients under her care. Hopefully this would not be pursued, until all other options have been explored.

–Shellie Simons

If I were to have a conversation with the nurse manager, I would first ask what she believes is the right thing to do for Lori. We would discuss how Lori is handling the accident and how Lori feels about this situation. I would ask if employee assistance was offered to help Lori talk about her concerns related to what happened. Ultimately, I would be most concerned about whether Lori is going to be able to handle the situation mentally and emotionally.

Lori is focusing much of her energy on the care of her family, and these distractions have caused a patient to be harmed. I would ask if Lori has been offered family leave and, knowing Lori is so concerned about work, whether the organization offered her other options. Would she be willing to apply for PTO donations or investigate other opportunities for her to be paid while she is caring for her mother? I would also ask the nurse manager whether she provided Lori with the option of speaking with hospice or a social worker to assist with options in her mother's care. There are different agencies and support groups that are available to help.

As nurse leaders, we are responsible for creating a safe and healthy work environment for our patients and our staff. It is our responsibility to have conversations with our staff about caring for themselves and their patients. We don't always go beyond the initial obvious questions, however. When we ask a question, we need to ensure we are addressing all the issues underlying the answers provided.

In this situation, as with many, I am not sure that the nurse manager really asked all the right questions. The organization did not seem to offer Lori assistance with the one thing that she needed, which was dealing with her financial concerns. An effective leader asks the probing questions to assist the staff in making the best decision.

When an adverse event like this happens, it is important to make sure the staff member involved is adequately prepared to handle this situation. Staff members involved may blame themselves, and it is important for them to know that you support them through this difficult time. While this is a horrible situation, we need to use this as a learning opportunity and encourage Lori not to blame herself for this incident.

–Patti Hart

Reflection

While some nurse managers are open to hearing about their employees' personal lives, others would prefer to keep their work and home lives separate. This will inevitably influence how the manager deals with worrisome behaviors among his/her staff. Think of a personal issue a worker shared with you and how comfortable you were in dealing with it. In hindsight, do you wish you had responded differently? If so, how?

Would you describe yourself as "best buddies" or "strictly business" with those who work for you, and how does this impact your ability to handle personal and lifestyle issues?

Summary

While the guidelines for professional behavior during work hours are often spelled out in endless policies, many nurse managers find themselves struggling to deal with the increasingly porous boundary between on- and off-the-job behavior. In particular, technology can offer both quick and accurate information as well as destructive and damaging rumors. Often, the concept of "privacy" is replaced by "transparency."

Regardless of your management style, the people you supervise need to know what your expectations are. Do you want them to come to you if they are struggling with personal crises? Are you opposed to staff members using their cell phones for personal calls when there is a slow time at work? At a staff meeting, discuss how personal situations should be handled when they impact work performance, and poll your employees for their thoughts.

For many reasons—including legal ones—communicating with your staff about these issues is essential. Take a position and stick with it, but be prepared to hold yourself to the same standard of behavior. Chiding a nurse for surfing the Internet for shoes is unfair if you do the same thing in the privacy of your office.

Activity

Watch or talk about an episode or clip of the television show *Nurse Jackie*. Reflect on the following questions:

- Do you have an obligation to address your coworkers' well-being?

- Would you go to a higher authority if Nurse Jackie were your coworker? If so, who?

Controlling personal stress is an important strategy. Find an online stress inventory (there are several at www.health education.uci.edu/stress/stressinventory.aspx), take it, and think about the following:

- Do you ever struggle with balancing personal and professional aspects of your life?

- What are your coping strategies when stressed?

- Do you think you're more or less stressed than your coworkers?

Consider having your staff perform these same activities.

part III i'm not ok, and neither are you

8 | the murse

For some, nursing is a quintessentially female endeavor. Yet in its survey of registered nurses in 2008, the U.S. Department of Health and Human Services found that the number of male nurses (which we affectionately call "murses") in the workforce is steadily increasing. In particular, the survey found:

> *In 2008, 6.6 percent of all RNs were male, a small increase from 5.8 percent in 2004. However, the share of male nurses was much higher for the more recent nursing graduates. Only 4.1 percent of nurses who graduated in 1990 or earlier were male, while 9.6 percent of those who completed their initial RN education after 1990 were male (U.S. Department of Health and Human Services, 2010, p.13).*

Increasing gender diversity among registered nurses is generally understood to be a positive move forward for the profession. In particular, as the patient population becomes increasingly diverse, it is beneficial to have variability in the demographic characteristics of our nursing force (Andrews, Stewart, Morgan, & D'Arcy, 2012). In other words, because a lot of our patients are male, it makes sense to have some male nurses. Interestingly, patients still seem to prefer female nurses—even some male patients.

Some aren't so sure that male nurses are good for nursing, though. Author Joan Evans argues that the growing number of men in the nursing profession is *not* a sign of progressive gender integration. Instead, she says, the increasing number of men in nursing serves only to disproportionally situate men in administrative and elite positions. Evans writes:

Male nurses do this by employing strategies that allow them to distance themselves from female colleagues and the quintessential feminine image of nursing itself, as a prerequisite to elevating their own prestige and power. They are aided in this task by patriarchal cultural institutions that create and perpetuate male advantage, as well as by women nurses themselves who, consciously or unconsciously, nurture the careers of men colleagues (Evans, 1997, p. 226).

Although we can hope that today—16 years later—this is not the predominant view of most women in nursing, it's safe to assume that many nurses still ascribe to this perspective. Unfortunately, the media often further reinforces stereotypes about "male nurses."

Gender stereotypes are pervasive for both male and female nurses. For some men, there may be an assumption that advancing up through the ranks is easier, or that men promote less drama on the unit, or that men have a "fix-it" style of management that does not always effectively deal with all the important variables in a situation.

In the magazine *Scrubs: The Nurse's Guide to Good Living*, Jim DeMaria articulates three male nurse myths:

- **Nursing is a woman's profession:** There is a sense among some that the care profession is only for women. This perspective, however, is slowly (very slowly!) changing. It is becoming more accepted for men to be in traditionally female roles, such as nursing.

- **Men aren't emotionally suited to nursing:** Some folks believe that the fix-it attitude held by some men doesn't jive well with the overall purpose and goals of nursing. However, a concrete, ends-oriented approach can often be a welcome addition to a care team.

- **Male nurses are just "wannabe" doctors.** This myth is perhaps the most demeaning toward nursing as a profession. The idea that the only reason a man would become a nurse is because he's a wannabe doctor reduces the profession of nursing to something that is less-than and second-best (DeMaria, 2011).

Each of these myths was perhaps born from a kernel of truth. Regardless, male nurses have to fight against these misconceptions every day.

Research does support the idea that there are differences between male and female nurses. Male RNs are more likely to report that they have seen attractive nursing job opportunities and that they have looked for other employment within the past year than their female counterparts. Male RNs are also more likely than female RNs to report having experienced a threat of assault, emotional abuse, verbal or sexual harassment, or sexual assault while at work. There are, however, probably more similarities than differences between male and female nurses. Both have similar perceptions of job security, work flexibility, and ease of finding a new job (Andrews et al., 2012).

Vignettes, Commentaries, and Reflective Thinking

The remainder of this chapter presents vignettes about the murse, commentaries about the experiences represented in the vignettes, and opportunities to explore or reflect on the material.

Vignette 8.1: Male Drama

Cynthia is new to the OR but has worked on other units throughout the hospital. On the first day of real work after orientation, she has coffee with Ginny, a longtime OR nurse. "You'll like it here," Ginny says, after hearing about some of the problems with "drama" that Cynthia experienced on other floors. "There are more men, so it's not so high maintenance, if you know what I mean."

"I sure do!" Cynthia replies. "Women are so bitchy. I got to the point where I just couldn't stand it anymore. I'm glad for the change in environment."

Expert Commentary: Vignette 8.1

Change the setting and the names, and this could be a conversation had by many practicing nurses over the course of their careers. In my own career, I was welcomed into and celebrated by an all-female RN critical-care unit as the first male nurse to practice in the unit in many years. Men are welcomed more and more into nursing not only because of their physical strength to assist in patient care but more so for their positive effect on the unit culture. They also bring a unique perspective on how to relate to one another and solve problems. However, this can be a very sensitive issue for men to discuss in wide circles of peers due to the "sexist" label that can quickly be applied to male nurses who openly discuss it.

Shifting from a perspective of "better than" to one of "different from," while learning to value that difference and hold the conversation, is an important area of development for the nursing profession. The conversation has to start from a place of authenticity, focusing on characteristics, values, and beliefs that create sameness in both genders in the profession and learning from the differences. Leaders can work toward creating an environment that encourages and allows for issues, concerns, and problems to be explored from both perspectives. This can be difficult for many leaders, as it requires a shift in our own stereotypical mental models and being open to different ways of leading. Informal work groups, balanced between male and female, to strengthen the valuing and understanding of all perspectives.

It is important to realize that we can overgeneralize in situations based on our backgrounds, experiences, and beliefs. Welcoming new people into your unit is important, but avoid negatively coloring their initial experiences with your own. Let new people experience the culture and make their own decisions. Additionally, it's not OK to make stereotypical remarks about gender in either direction. Give and demand respect from your colleagues regarding both genders and don't tolerate gender-biased comments.

–Cole Edmonson

The modern workplace is a very diverse environment. Employees as individuals, both male and female, come from various racial and ethnic backgrounds. In this vignette, the protagonist says that the new nurse will like being in the OR because there are more male than female nurses, which she translates into "less drama." It is important to be cautious with the stereotyping occurring here. Personal experience reveals that although working with all male nurses down a particular wing or in a unit on occasion seemed to be more relaxing at times, there were also plenty of pleasant shifts spent working with all female colleagues. The point to remember is that they are all colleagues and should be treated as such. Treat others how one would like to be treated, and expect the same in return, no more and certainly no less. There will be times on the unit or floor when the environment seems more charged or the day is more stressful. It is usually not the makeup of the male-to-female nurse ratio, however, that causes this, but rather multiple factors such as case mix, patient acuity, staffing levels, patient-family interactions with staff, and unpredictable emergent issues that really add to the "drama."

–Eric Messner

Reflection

When comparing male and female approaches to conflict, how can a nurse manager be sensitive to differences without stereotyping?

Many women believe working with men eliminates drama in their professional lives. How does this play out at your organization? What skill sets, if any, seem to be more common in men?

Vignette 8.2: ManageMan

Jack was a nurse manager before becoming a nursing supervisor at Mercy Hospital. He has a "fix-it" approach to problems that sometimes causes conflicts. For example, Judy, an RN on L&D, came to Jack with a problem about one of her coworkers, who was calling off frequently. After a minute of explanation, Jack cut Judy off. "You've done everything you need to do," Jack said. "She's fired."

"But she's having a lot of personal problems, and I think that's what is underlying her call-offs," Judy answers, ready to explore alternatives to help the nurse in question.

"Tell her to get a therapist," Jack replies.

Another time, Jack arbitrarily pulled one nurse from the medical floor and sent her to the surgical floor without consulting the nurse manager of either unit. "They needed help. I got it for them," he explained to the director of nursing, who received a complaint after the incident.

Expert Commentary: Vignette 8.2

The "fix-it" mentality is not solely a male characteristic. It is, in fact, shared by both sexes and seems to be more person and leadership-style dependent. Leaders of both sexes who approach opportunities with this mentality generally get the same poor to fair results, especially if this is their preferred approach to all issues. However, being quick to action is valued in many situations in health care, especially where patient safety is concerned. Nevertheless, even quick-to-action situations need to be debriefed for learning and future applications.

Nurse leaders have different tolerance levels for mediocrity and ambiguity that are not necessarily based on their gender but more on their early development as leaders. In nursing, we find ourselves often wanting to "fix" situations, problems, and people. It is an element of our education and training as nurses, using clinical deductive reasoning methodologies to identify issues to which we apply our clinical knowledge base to correct or "fix." Simply moving into management positions does not shift that mental model. We often continue to want to "fix" people—not just patients, but also staff and unit situations. It's less clinical and more managerial. Revisiting our foundational knowledge in psychology and sociology can quickly remind us managers that we cannot "fix" people or situations, as we are not in control. Instead, we have moved into the role of influencer.

Managers can set the conditions for successful change by providing wisdom, knowledge, expectations, education, and resources needed for the individual or group to make the change. For a successful change process to occur, one must realize that nursing is a collective profession that does value the individual, but generally not at the expense of the group conformity. Being clear on the difference between managing processes and systems and leading people may help the leader refocus on being the facilitator of change and solutions, as opposed to the decision-maker using formal power to resolve the situation. The less the leader uses formal power, and the more the leader creates a group competent in creating its own solutions within the guardrails, the better the solution and the better prepared the group will be for solving future issues. Leaders must allow for the human condition. However, this cannot prevent a leader from acting.

It is important to remember that we, as leaders, must be sensitive to people and situations we are managing. Our leadership style needs to be flexible, or contingent. Respecting confidentiality as a manager in situations regarding employee performance needs to be of primary importance. Managers making comments to staff regarding other staff's performance or status in the organization not only violates confidentiality norms but also disrespects the individual involved. It is not a characteristic of leaders who must protect this information and safeguard employee rights.

–Cole Edmonson

A "fix-it" or reactionary orientation may be necessary to solve an immediate or emergent issue, like multiple traumas coming into the emergency department from a multivehicle collision. If this is employed as an everyday management style, however, conflicts may arise. Some problems can be averted or avoided altogether when a more open, receptive, and proactive management style is employed. Proactive managers can often anticipate certain "expected" issues and develop and implement measures designed to mitigate or ease their impact. In the case of the emergency department laden with incoming traumas, a proactive manager may have an on-call pool of nurses in place for times when patient surge surpasses the capacity of the staff to provide adequate care. There is no crystal ball or prescribed rules of engagement, but forward-thinking management styles will often result in fewer conflicts (and complaints) and in having measures in place to deal with conflicts when they occur.

In this vignette, a nurse faces the possibility of being summarily fired without being offered an opportunity to explain her actions. Summary dismissals are rare occurrences, usually reserved for grievous actions. There needs to be more open dialogue and a fact-finding process, as there may be more to the story or extenuating circumstances. Most institutions have employee-assistance programs available, and it may be wiser to assist a struggling employee through a period of strife than to be encumbered with the time and expense of training a new replacement. As for the other scenario discussed in the vignette, when moving nurses about the health care facility to accommodate staffing, it may be more efficient to consult with the specific floor managers to determine their immediate staffing requirements, as they are usually more informed as to specific shift-to-shift needs and what would be most beneficial for their particular unit. Furthermore, floating a medically oriented nurse to a surgical floor may place that nurse in an uncomfortable position, compromise patient care and safety, and be unnecessary if more appropriate resources are available.

–Eric Messner

Reflection

Conflict resolution styles vary with the degree and type of problem being confronted. How would your colleagues describe your management style? How about your staff?

How does the predominance of men in supervisory and administrative positions create tension? What strategies have you used to address the inverse pyramid of power that has occurred in nursing?

Vignette 8.3: Through the Ranks

Sacred Heart Hospital has an opening for a nurse manager in the OR. Several longtime RNs apply for the position, as does Glenn, a nurse with limited experience but a BSN and graduate coursework in nursing administration. After 2 weeks of deliberation, Glenn is offered the job.

This infuriates the three other RNs who applied. They are female and more experienced. "You know, you only got that job because you're a man," one of them tells Glenn.

"Yeah," says another. "Men in nursing get opportunities more often, just because they're guys."

Glenn starts to explain his educational background, but the nurses walk away, still complaining to each other. For months thereafter, the three "rejected" RNs do everything they can to sabotage Glenn's work performance.

Expert Commentary: Vignette 8.3

Let's start with the real issue: anger and resentment over a less-experienced nurse getting a promotion over a more-experienced one. Without knowing the degrees of the other three candidates, it's difficult to determine whether that was a factor. In general, however, the BSN adds a management competency that is not always learned through clinical experience or in associate degree programs.

Despite the generalization by the three female candidates, no studies exist to this author's knowledge that demonstrate a correlation between being male and garnering promotions in nursing. Men often gravitate toward leadership opportunities as their own career goals, but often they are encouraged by their female counterparts to pursue these opportunities as well.

Regardless of how or why Glenn got the job, he won't be able to talk his way logically out of the situation, as it appears to be influenced by emotional bias. The facts are the facts, but logic rarely wins over emotion.

Sabotage for any reason in the clinical setting is not only destructive to the professional practice environment, but it also endangers patient safety, directly and indirectly. Glenn needs to confront the situation head-on with the support of his supervisor and possibly of human-resources professionals. Behavior is one of the most difficult dimensions of performance to deal with in individuals in the health care environment, but one of the most important. Health care is not just about tasks and interventions; it is predicated on relationships and communication that are both complex and critical to outcomes. Disruptive behavior in health care environments is a large and unacceptable deterrent to the critical process of professional communication that needs to occur to keep patients and providers safe from harm.

As a leader, you must document, document, and document again the behavior, confront it directly, and explore with each individual his or her motivations, including past experiences. Then, you must set the expectation of positive behavior and gain the person's commitment to corrective actions going forward, while also holding him or her accountable for those actions. Remember, when leaders do not take the needed actions to correct or address negative, destructive behavior of individuals or groups on a unit, it will eventually reflect on the leader and diminish his or her ability to lead effectively. In other words, the leader's credibility will decrease with the group he or she is supposed to lead and potentially with colleagues as well.

Passive-aggressive behavior and sabotage—two significant themes in this vignette—have no place in the health care setting. These two behaviors undermine positive professional relationships and can create unsafe situations for staff and patients. Time and energy spent on these destructive behaviors take focus away from patient care, patient safety, and surveillance, and decrease employee engagement.

–Cole Edmonson

There is a trend in the nursing profession to continually advance ourselves—in our art, our science, and our clinical practice. It's what nurses do. Twenty years ago, bedside nursing consisted of registered nurses (RNs) and licensed practical nurses (LPNs) working side by side to provide patient care. But health care and technology constantly change, as does the required skill set. The baccalaureate wave began, as did the push to hire nurses with advanced degrees. Licensed practical nurses moved away from hospital-based nursing care, even though many LPNs initially had far more experience than their baccalaureate-trained replacements. The trend toward completing higher levels of education continues today, with the baccalaureate degree looked upon as the minimum required entry point for hospital-based RN nursing care. Advanced practice nurses are likewise affected by the cries for higher education, usually completing degrees at the master's preparatory level as a bare minimum. In addition, there are calls for upcoming advanced practice clinicians to be prepared at the doctoral level in the not-so-distant future.

The trend will likely continue, as nurses continually evolve the discipline of nursing. It is not surprising, then, for this newly hired nurse manager to have garnered some resentment from more-experienced nurses who believed they were better candidates. What they failed to appreciate was that his baccalaureate training and graduate coursework in nursing administration may better prepare him to be a successful nurse manager. The recommendation for all staff members is to maximize their education and potential, especially if a career in nursing administration is desired. In some institutions, master's-level preparation is the new minimum requirement for all nurse managers. The trend for nursing leadership—male or female—is moving toward attaining advanced degrees and pursuing continuing education as our nursing art, science, and practice evolve.

–Eric Messner

Reflection

Given the tendency for men to be overt and women to be covert in expressing conflict, how do you adjust your management style to accommodate problem solving and crisis management?

Since medicine has traditionally been a male profession, what dynamics do you see occurring between men who are nurses and physicians who are male?

How can you, as nurse manager, encourage your staff to be open-minded and nonjudgmental in an institution that may not be diverse in terms of gender or culture?

Vignette 8.4: Sexism

Dave works on a medical-surgical floor and rotates days and nights. Last week, he was working a predictably quiet night shift with Sandy and Tiffany. At one point in the evening, Dave walked into the staff room as Sandy was showing Tiffany a "Sexiest Man Alive" magazine cover. Sandy said, "Wowie, look at that jawline! Man, I would sure love to see him in a pair of biker shorts!"

Dave didn't say anything to them, and the comment didn't bother him, but he thought to himself, "What a double standard! If another male nurse and I had been ogling a picture of a scantily clad beautiful woman and making objectifying remarks, my female colleagues would have been pretty upset."

Expert Commentary: Vignette 8.4

Dave could not be more right. Double standards are everywhere in our world, including health care. Is it right? No! Is it the world we sometimes live in? Yes! From a human-resources perspective, there's really no difference in the situations; both are not part of what we expect in health care. However, the egregiousness of the situation is probably predicated on the people involved, how they feel about it, and whether it meets their threshold of personal tolerance for sexual innuendo, harassment, or inappropriateness.

Basically, three paths exist for Dave:

- Report the incident to human resources or a supervisor.

- If he wasn't offended, ignore it and see if it becomes a trend.

- Talk to the colleagues who made the remarks in front of him.

You can't go wrong with taking the third approach. Sometimes, just bringing the double-standard issue to your colleagues' awareness can cause their behavior to change. We operate from our own perspectives and are ethnocentric in our views; although uncomfortable, most people will appreciate being gently reminded there are numerous perspectives in the world, especially the small world of a nursing unit.

Just because it doesn't bother Dave doesn't mean it's OK. Many such norms exist in society and depend on gender, race, belief systems, backgrounds, culture, and even the area you live in. We can become desensitized to these double standards such that they no longer even meet our threshold to cause us to act. Gaining perspective from a colleague who doesn't share your belief system or norms is a good place to start to learn about the differences between people, but more importantly, how we are the same.

–Cole Edmonson

Double standards abound in life. However it is understandable that a male nurse might take offense to the comments he overheard. In today's workplace, there has to be a collegiality toward our coworkers, and employees should be cautioned to err on the side of professionalism. These days, a culture of sensitivity and diversity is the expectation and the norm. Everyone has to work together. Comments like the ones in the vignette have no place in the work environment.

–Eric Messner

Reflection

How do you, as nurse manager, encourage a professional attitude, even during downtimes at work?

Is there a policy about sexist behavior at your institution? Should there be? What would it look like?

What would you have done if you had walked in on a situation similar to the one above?

Vignette 8.5: The Nurse Is a Man

Simon is an excellent nurse, and most days he really enjoys his job. Simon is taking care of a difficult postsurgical patient who demands a lot of his time. Simon has been responding to this patient's call bell all day, so when it goes off again, he is not surprised. He goes into the room and discovers that the patient has evacuated her bowels. Simon goes to clean the patient up, and the patient cries, "No! I need a *real* nurse this time!"

Simon is extremely frustrated, but leaves the room to try to find a "real" nurse, which he interprets to be female. The only available person is Caroline, who is pretty old school. Caroline enters the patient's room and says, "Well, of course I can understand why you wouldn't want Simon to help you with this particular problem."

Simon is exasperated. He thinks to himself, "I have to work with this patient for the rest of the day. My nurse colleague has just undercut me to the patient, which is going to make my job so much harder!"

Expert Commentary: Vignette 8.5

First, let's be clear that men are "real" nurses. Many stereotypes exist regarding what makes a real nurse and about men who go into nursing, but that does not make them right or true. We do have to realize that there are female patients who clearly prefer to be cared for and examined by female providers—not just female nurses but physicians as well. It is their right to choose who cares for them in a respectful way that is not based on prejudice, just as nurses have the right to refuse to participate in care that violates their personal moral philosophies or religious beliefs.

Being male nurses, we need to be sensitive toward all our patients, especially female patients, who may be uncomfortable with certain intimate aspects of care being provided by male nurses. Generally, it's not personal toward the male nurse; it's more personal for the patient. Offering the patients options and not assuming they are comfortable with care that exposes the genitalia to the opposite sex is always a good practice. Maintaining that sensitivity is always a good practice for any nurse, regardless of gender.

Patients don't deserve, nor should they be exposed to, a nurse's bias, especially at a time when they are most vulnerable. The destruction of the patient-nurse relationship with comments regarding preconceived notions, derogatory comments, and comments furthering prejudice is, in fact, unprofessional behavior. Every nurse should feel comfortable and obligated to have a crucial conversation with a colleague who makes such comments. When we accept or permit the behavior, we are in fact promoting it.

In summary, be sensitive to the patients you are caring for. Just because you may be comfortable performing the task doesn't mean your patient is comfortable with you doing it. When patients want to talk about a nurse colleague, it's OK to listen, but you must find something to "manage up" about your colleague. Don't perpetuate negative stereotypes that come from patients. Lastly, professionally confront colleagues regarding negative, nonproductive comments about you or other colleagues. Think of it this way: If a patient were going to harm himself or herself, you would be obligated to intervene. This is really no different: Your colleague is harming the unit environment, harming relationships, and perpetuating stereotypes—and no good can come of it.

–Cole Edmonson

There are lots of different ways to look at this situation, but perhaps the best way is to identify the areas where miscommunication may have occurred. What did the patient mean by "real" nurse? What were Simon's perceptions of a "real" nurse? What were Simon's expectations of Caroline when he requested her assistance? In acquiescing to the patient's request and finding another nurse to complete the task, Simon has already undercut himself. He was complying with the patient's request, but it might have been better for Simon to ask for partial assistance to help complete the task himself.

Demanding or difficult patients will be part of every nurse's career. Sometimes, ground rules must be set with these patients. By seeking Caroline's assistance, Simon may have led the patient to assume that he wasn't up to the task. Caroline's comments to the patient may have reinforced this perception.

After a situation like this one, it's a good idea to conduct a debriefing session. During this session, the nurse manager could encourage staff to work together to accomplish tasks, but leave the primary nurse in charge to provide direct care for his or her patient. Staff must be reminded to be respectful of each other and avoid disparaging comments that may undercut the credibility of other staff or personnel when talking with patients or their family members. Situations may arise when personality differences between staff and patients necessitate reassignment of staff to meet difficult patient demands in a more discerning manner.

–Eric Messner

Reflection

How could this situation be avoided so that all nurses on the unit felt supported and valued?

Do you "manage up," providing staff with respect for their abilities at the same time as you challenge them to a higher standard?

Summary

Interestingly, the gender status quo seems to be continuing in nursing, making it unlikely that nursing will follow the trend of medicine and become an equally attractive profession for men and women. (Our current mix of medical students is divided almost equally, with perhaps a percentage point or two favoring women.) That being said, all nurses are nurses: They've taken the same licensure exam and been hired into the same job descriptions. Therefore, debates about the legitimacy of "male nurses" should be a nonissue.

The tolerant workplace is a compliant workplace, preventing litigation before discrimination can occur. Acceptance and inclusion begin with you, the nurse manager. As those you lead observe your interactions with others who may be different in terms of gender or cultural background, they will have an example of desired behavior. Regular visuals (posters, resource books, and scholarly articles) as well as spoken reinforcements will demonstrate your values in concrete and tangible ways.

A nurse manager's ability to promote a tolerant workplace is only as good as the higher-ups in administration. Among your peers, a similar ethic of acceptance and support should be modeled as a guideline for others, and policies toward enforcement should be developed. Reporting of incidents needs to occur promptly on both a unit and organizational level. Remember, health care providers work as a team, and you are the leader of that team.

Activity

Interview two nurses who are men, preferably from outside your organization. (Online forums are a great option for this. A Google search on 11/26/12 revealed a great post with 140 comments at www.nursetogether.com, titled "I Am a Male Nurse.")

Ask the following questions:

- Do you think there's a fundamental difference between male and female nurses?

- What's it like to be a nurse who is male in a profession that is primarily female?

- What have you experienced during your nursing career that you feel is unique to your gender?

Use the information to identify some key insights that you can then share within your own institution.

9 | better than you

Nursing is a profession of many hierarchies. There are perceptions about which educational degree prepares you best for the clinical setting, as well as thoughts about the superiority of certain areas of practice, with the more acute usually ranked the highest. With so many avenues into nursing, longevity seems to be less important than in the past, although it, too, can play a role.

While "rankism" can help workers understand a bit of the social order in any setting, for nurses, this practice can lead to fractured care and frustration. Believing that you are not as good as the other nurses you work with can become a self-fulfilling prophecy as well as a recipe for lowered self-esteem, depression, and a host of other problems.

Some examples of nurse rankism include the following:

- Viewing a float nurse as *persona non grata*. Often, the permanent nurses won't talk to float nurses beyond what is required and give them the worst assignments.

- One or more nurses feel superior to others because of age, experience, or education, and act as if it's an imposition to work with those of "lesser abilities."

- International nurses are misunderstood and mistreated.

- Members of one unit believe they are better than those of another—for example, ICU versus the medical-surgical ward or hospital nurses versus those employed in long-term care or rehabilitation.

- An individual with a superiority complex and a position of status (perhaps a nurse manager) lets others know they are not as accomplished and able as he or she is.

Fuller (2010) encourages managers to promote an understanding and appreciation for the role of all coworkers, noting the need to treat all nurses with dignity in order to create a harmonious workplace. He also suggests that health care providers, in particular, treat their clients (i.e., patients) as partners and that doctors, especially, need to set aside ego.

Ellingston (2002) suggests that health care teams exist along a continuum, with some having loose coordination and others tight. The ultimate in teamwork is synergistic teamwork, where different disciplines come together without regard for the status of each member. She notes that perceptions of teamwork increase with one's professional status, so that physicians are much more likely to believe they are working as a team than support staff. She points out that with nurse practitioners performing some of the same functions as a physician, the blurring of boundaries can be threatening. Ultimately, the best teams work together with give-and-take on the part of all members, as opposed to a paternalistic team when one member is "in charge."

McCloughen, O'Brien, and Jackson (2009) interviewed 13 nurse leaders and discovered that in contrast to using senior status as a kind of weapon against coworkers, being mentored by a senior nurse early in their career was a pivotal process. In fact, those mentored felt they wouldn't have become leaders without such mentorship. The themes these authors discovered in the interviews on becoming a leader reveal much about the power of nurses supporting nurses: considering each other with positive regard, developing respectful boundaries, and honoring key human characteristics.

Within the nursing hierarchies, jealousy and competition can often add another layer of conflict. Susan Shapiro Barash (2006) interviewed women from diverse backgrounds and reports that competition between women is often covert but cruel. She suggests that women are trained from an early age to view competition as sexual and negative. While men have "rivalries," women are "jealous." Nurses shared stories with us about this dynamic: A younger, more attractive nurse is favored, and those who advance up the career ladder often are viewed with a mixture of admiration and resentment.

Gray (2012) learned that women feel more jealousy and envy toward other women than they do toward men. In contrast, men do not feel the same way about each other. She pointed out that women need "allies" at work, especially in higher-ranking positions, but they have trouble finding them for this very reason. Even appearance has an impact. Studies have shown that women who provide pictures of themselves with job applications are less likely to be hired if they are unattractive or overweight. The question becomes, how do we help women get along when they feel threatened by their peers? Our commentators suggest several alternatives.

Carol Tringali said this about the situation:

The leader/staff nurse colleague relationship can be compromised because of poor communication and lack of appreciation of the value of each person's contribution toward the end result of safe, efficient patient care. Communication, in its most comprehensive definition, is important in the development of relationships. Such communication involves active listening, compassion, and empathy.

She continues:

It is a two-way exchange of ideas that results in both people understanding the situation or the other person's perspective better. With better understanding, movement to mutually satisfying actions/solutions can be achieved. Colleagues then become engaged with each other in the pursuit of a common goal, i.e., patient care.

While women are learning to compete in healthy ways, there is still room for improvement. The greater the acceptance of each nurse for the abilities he or she brings to the workplace, the better collaboration and patient care.

Maybe it's time nurses started playing golf together or forming sports teams to learn what men seem to have mastered long ago: Competition doesn't have to destroy relationships. In fact, it might improve them.

Vignettes, Commentaries, and Reflective Thinking

The remainder of this chapter presents vignettes about hierarchies, social order, and perceptions; commentaries about the experiences represented in the vignettes; and opportunities to explore or reflect on the material.

Vignette 9.1: Superiority Complex

Rose, a "mature" nurse, takes great pride in being the most experienced employee on the geriatric unit. Whenever a new nurse appears on the unit, Rose goes to great lengths to tell him or her that she has been at Grace Hospital since the unit opened.

One busy day on the unit, Tammy, a float nurse who regularly comes to the geriatric unit, is assigned to work with Rose. As soon as Tammy arrives, Rose gives an exaggerated sigh. "Oh gosh, I guess I'll have to help you all day—again," she says to Tammy, who thinks she's joking and laughs.

Rose spends most of the morning telling Tammy how to do even basic procedures that Tammy is competent to perform alone. Eventually, Tammy feels as if Rose is condescending and trying to give her the message she's just not good enough to work on the geriatric unit. "Just because she's been here 20 years doesn't mean she's better than me," Tammy tells the supervisor. "Please, don't send me there again."

Expert Commentary: Vignette 9.1

Rankism is about putting someone down to elevate the status of one's self—a matter of poor self-esteem. Its roots are in envy of another as well as in the power inherent in hierarchical structure. If a pecking order on a nursing unit does exist, it's usually because there is a self-appointed leader. It's helpful to keep in mind that floors and units are also cultures, often with a cliquish nature. Cliques always reject those who are not members, and outsider is a common position for float nurses like Tammy. The verbal attacks, persistent put-downs in front of others, and sarcasm create a hostile work environment for Tammy and can damage her in unseen ways, including her personal health. Zero tolerance for assaults on another's self-esteem would be an appropriate policy. A courageous dialogue with Rose is in order.

Generational issues are at play here. More importantly, because Tammy has informed the supervisor of her experiences on the unit, an appropriate and accountable action is to write about the incident, keep notes for future reference and upcoming evaluations, and consult with HR.

A facilitated meeting with Tammy and Rose is also in order. It helps to set rules of engagement agreed to by all parties before each shares her perspective. Tammy is the authority on how she feels, so using "I" messages such as "I feel [mad/ hurt, frustrated/humiliated] about [specific, observable behavior] because [impact of behavior]." Rose can also have a chance to explain, clarify, or even apologize if she is clueless about how she is perceived in this situation.

The supervisor has a teachable human-resources moment to review the hospital's values, policies, and consequences for any individual who creates a hostile environment, which can negatively affect patient care, teamwork, and organizational performance. Speaking of education, Tammy would benefit from an assertiveness class, and Rose could use a class on bullying/ lateral violence in the workplace. The whole unit needs further in-service training as well.

–G. Rumay Alexander

Rose, through her tenure, perceives herself as the expert nurse on the geriatric unit. This elite self-designation sets the stage for a work environment in which bullying or insidious intimidation can flourish. Rose may perceive a threat to her position and status and has resorted to classic bullying behaviors to maintain her influence—unwarranted criticism and excessive monitoring of a competent and experienced nurse. It is also likely that Rose will exhibit the same behavior with other nurses if she continues to feel a threat to her status on the unit. Tammy reacts in a manner that relieves the problem for her by requesting not to work again on the unit with Rose. However, this does not eliminate the problem that Rose's behavior creates for the unit and the ability to ensure the recruitment and retention of qualified staff. On the surface, Rose's behavior may be seen as benign, but for the recipient of Rose's unnecessary attention, the behavior is seen as intimidation and bullying. Once the nurse manager is made aware of the situation, she can continue to assess the ongoing impact of Rose's behavior on the unit.

–M.T. Meadows

In this vignette, Tammy voices to her supervisor that there is an issue between her and Rose. Instead of simply agreeing with Tammy's request to not be sent to that unit again, Tammy's supervisor could offer to support and mentor Tammy, so she can assert herself with Rose. As a first step, the supervisor could show Tammy how she can acknowledge Rose's notable expertise while at the same time asserting herself as a competent nurse. For example, Tammy could mention to Rose that she does not need to take it upon herself to take time out of her busy schedule to help with tasks that Tammy feels competent performing on her own, but at the same time that Tammy feels privileged and reassured that someone with Rose's expertise could be counted on if she were to ask for help or support.

Tammy's supervisor could also verify whether other nurses from the floating team have had similar experiences with Rose. If so, she could offer to support and mentor them to also assert themselves with Rose. The supervisor may also decide to discuss the issue with Rose's supervisor to inform her that while Rose may mean well, the way some of her peers perceive Rose's actions is in fact tarnishing the unit's reputation and leading to some nurses not wanting to work on that unit anymore.

–Isabelle St-Pierre

Reflection

When one nurse feels a need to project a "superiority complex" on others, he or she usually has an agenda that is not about improving the work product of her peers. How can you, the nurse manager, help such nurses feel more secure about their abilities?

What do you believe to be the dividing line between helpful feedback and overbearing and unwarranted criticism? How do you navigate that line?

Vignette 9.2: Taking Advantage

Bess, a PRN nurse on the medical floor of Kingdom Hospital, hates to work with Sherry, who deliberately gives her the worst patients to care for. "I'm here to help, not be abused," she tells Sherry, after she is assigned to care for eight difficult patients while the regular nurses have only seven. Sherry just shrugs her shoulders and tells Bess if she doesn't want to be sent to their floor, someone else will do the work.

Joan, one of the regular nurses, tells Bess that Sherry criticized her work the last time she was assigned to the medical floor. "Sherry said the hospital wouldn't hire you full time because you couldn't handle the heat," Joan confides. "That's why she loaded you up with all the patients we had to give extra time and energy to yesterday."

Expert Commentary: Vignette 9.2

"What You Should Do When You Are Set Up to Fail" could be the title of this vignette. Emotions run on high when "hate" is on the scene. Recognize that passive-aggressive behavior is at work and can quite easily go unnoticed by others. Where the implicit is not made explicit, injustices flourish. Joan's comments—while informative—only add fuel to the fire.

For the immediate situation, Bess has the right to say she is willing to accept her fair share of the workload, but that in her opinion, patient safety could be compromised; hence, she is respectfully asking for alterations in the assignment. This discussion is best held with witnesses present—in particular, Joan. This is a situation in which *what* is said is just as important as *how* something is said. When emotions are running high, one's hearing is affected, and misunderstandings often arise. The use of a soft tone of voice and a moderate pace can be most effective. If the request is blown off and no changes occur, then it's appropriate for Beth to notify the shift supervisor.

Make the implicit explicit with documentation of the practices in question. Bess could ask Joan if she is willing to share with the supervisor either in person or in writing what Sherry said. Separate the public humiliation from the patient care issue and deal with this matter in a second notification to the supervisor. A meeting among all parties involved to further understand what is beneath the personal attack is warranted. Review the institution's policies regarding appreciative leadership components.

–G. Rumay Alexander

It is a long-term and chronic complaint of float nurses that they are given the "worst" assignments. In this vignette, both Sherry's action and her subsequent comment exhibit bullying behavior. Bess's complaint about the patient assignment was an opportunity for Sherry to assess the situation and adjust the assignment to ensure an equitable distribution of workload. However, through Sherry's responsibility for the patient assignment and her response when questioned, it is clear that Sherry exhibited bullying behavior: assigning an unrealistic workload and making derogatory comments. The subsequent comment from Joan, while appearing to be one of support, in actuality is continuation of the bullying behavior and culture of the unit. Gossiping on both the part of Sherry and Joan supports and strengthens a culture of lateral violence.

The nurse manager may not be aware of this behavior due to generalized peer acceptance and intimidation or a generalized attitude of "this is not my issue nor my fight." The nurse manager has the responsibility to ensure competent and safe care.

Staff rounding is one way to elicit feedback from the nursing staff. This "purposeful" rounding creates an open environment where problems are identified and addressed in real time.

–M.T. Meadows

This vignette is a perfect example of how, if she chose to intervene constructively, the action of a peer could potentially influence and even improve a difficult situation. In the second sentence, we see Bess trying to assert herself with Sherry by stating her discomfort with the patient assignment—albeit not in the most productive way. However, Sherry totally dismisses Bess's complaint and even belittles her. Instead of telling Bess what Sherry has said about her, Joan (who is an impartial third party privy to this deplorable situation) could instead decide to privately speak to Sherry about her concerns with her actions. Joan could point out to Sherry that it doesn't get anyone anywhere if she thinks Bess can't "handle the heat" and yet provides her with patient assignments that are far more difficult than those of regular nurses, who are probably better equipped to manage such a workload. Joan could also indicate to Sherry that she is in fact putting patients at risk and dampening the work climate by introducing resentment between the regular nurses and Bess. Joan could also ask Sherry to clarify her intentions. Why is she setting up Bess to fail?

If her intervention with Sherry is not successful, Joan could decide to bring the issue to her unit manager. She could tell the manager that she is concerned that Sherry's actions could be detrimental both to patients (by jeopardizing their safety) and staff (by negatively affecting the work climate and the reputation of the unit). When Joan talks with the manager, she can describe the steps she took to try to improve the situation (i.e., she already spoke with Sherry regarding the issue). The manager should then investigate the situation by interviewing Sherry and possibly Bess (either together or separately). This will provide the opportunity to clearly state her expectations to Sherry while outlining the consequences if they are not met. She can follow up in a few weeks to ensure that the situation is resolved.

–Isabelle St-Pierre

Reflection

Sociologists study in- and out-group behavior. At many hospitals, "out-groups" are part-timers and per diem nurses, with the full-time or regular workers becoming a de facto in-group. How do you help your staff avoid cliquish "in-group" behaviors and promote teamwork among all nurses? If you know of a clique that exists in your unit, what, if anything can you do to break it up?

Vignette 9.3: Global Issues

Southern California Hospital is a large hospital that employs a high percentage of Spanish-speaking nurses. The Spanish-speaking nurses talk to each other in Spanish all the time. As a result, the non-Spanish speakers band together and become upset and annoyed because they are automatically excluded from the conversation. The patients are also starting to complain because the nurses speak Spanish to each other in front of the patients. The patients feel like the nurses are talking about them in secret!

Expert Commentary: Vignette 9.3

The crux of the issue is below the surface of Spanish-speaking nurses talking to each other in Spanish. It is about what happens when cultures collide and differences surface. The frequently used iceberg metaphor best depicts this set of dynamics. Culture is like an iceberg. What is below the surface of the water is greater than the tip, which is highly visible. The tip in this case is language differences. All encounters are cultural encounters, and the importance of this fact is highly significant in the health care delivery environment.

When patients and providers come together, there are at least four cultures crashing into each other:

- The patient's culture
- The provider's culture

- The country's culture where the care is being given

- The organizational culture of the health care institution

The more differences between the provider and the patient, the more likely there will be points of friction. Also lying in the murky waters are power issues, trust issues, and fear. Those who are of the majority in terms of similarities have the power inherent in numbers and can make as well as enforce rules for those who are a minority. The overarching dynamic is our desire as humans to be comfortable. Given the changing demographics in this country, this scenario is becoming much more the norm.

Cultural appropriateness requires education. Health care institutions must be proactive and prepared for changes in their future. One method to stay on top of things is for leadership to conduct environmental scans at least every 6 months. The rapid changes of our world require strategic thinking and nimbleness in order to survive. Employee education regarding the Cultural and Linguistically Appropriate Standards (CLAS), language policies of the institution, and a review of the Joint Commission requirements for delivering culturally relevant care should be provided at orientation and incorporated in patient assessments and plans of care. If the institution declares English as the language to be used at all times, and those for whom English is not their primary language are hired, such declaration should be made known to applicants. English proficiency can be assessed along with provisions for language assistance if needed. Having bilingual providers is helpful and an asset in many situations, so it can be made clear that minimizing perceptions that create fear in patients is the primary goal. The dignity of all should be preserved.

–G. Rumay Alexander

Diversity in the health care workforce has increased along with the need for leadership skills to effectively manage a changing demographic. On the first review of this scenario, it is easy to identify that the Spanish-speaking nurses are exhibiting bullying behavior by communicating in a manner that withholds information from others and isolates patients from their caregivers.

The study of work group behaviors can offer a different explanation for the current situation. The Spanish-speaking nurses may perceive themselves to be a minority group within the unit team structure, resulting in feelings of inequality. Their resulting work behaviors may be a reaction to this perceived or real lack of control within the unit environment. The nurse manager needs to assess the situation to determine the root cause of this insidious intimidation on the unit. Is the behavior a result of a culture that does not value diversity? Regardless of the origins of the behavior, the nurse manager must act first to ensure that patients are cared for in a safe and effective manner. Unless the unit is employing a bilingual care model, it should be established that English must be used in communicating in the presence of nonbilingual patients and staff. The leadership work for the nurse manager then follows: responding to the issues of team behaviors and their etiology.

–M.T. Meadows

The challenges brought on by a diverse and multicultural workforce can be numerous. This vignette shows the importance for institutions to have clear policies pertaining to the language that employees are expected to use at work. As part of their general orientation, new employees must be made aware of the workplace policy pertaining to language expected to be used at work. Additionally, managers can remind their staff of this requirement on a regular basis, whether during a team meeting, via a memorandum or an email, or even informally when circulating on the unit. Managers can also remind staff that speaking the language dictated by the policy is also a way of showing respect and consideration for peers and patients who can then understand what is said between colleagues.

Managers may not necessarily be aware that employees are not communicating using the stipulated language. However, in this vignette, because patients were starting to complain, one can assume that the issue has been brought forward to the unit manager. The manager can therefore decide to address the issue broadly, for example as part of a team meeting, or speak directly to Spanish-speaking nurses to openly express his or her concerns. For example, the employees can be reminded that speaking in a foreign language in front of patients and/or peers who cannot understand the language is not only rude, but it in fact lacks professionalism and can create undue tension between people. Employees can also be reminded that patients who depend on health care professionals often feel very vulnerable and insecure, and they frequently perceive that every comment or discussion—especially in a language they cannot understand—is about them. As such, these patients may become suspicious and mistrusting of foreign nurses, potentially leading to a safety issue. Foreign nurses should be reminded that the fact that they can speak another language is not scorned but actually valued. They can even be encouraged to communicate in the language of choice of their patients (if they are able to do so). Conversely, they can be reminded to make a conscious effort to communicate in a language that will be understood by others while at work.

–Isabelle St-Pierre

Reflection

Nurse managers themselves may have their own beliefs and attitudes about health care. How does your ethnicity and/or gender influence your nursing practice?

When you need to raise awareness about a particular issue (such as speaking a language not everyone understands) are you more likely to open a dialogue with others or dictate in the form of a policy? Is one better than the other? Why?

Vignette 9.4: Shift Riff

Angie, the longtime evening nurse on a busy surgical floor, is in the midst of a feud with Erika, the longtime night nurse. The two nurses have been at each other for months, ever since a mistake was made on night shift that Erika believes was really Angie's fault.

Martha, a day nurse, fuels the flames between Angie and Erika by using shift report as a time to talk trash about each of them to the other. She tells Angie that rumors have been started about her inability to get all the work done on evening shift. The next morning, Erika complains to Martha about Angie accusing her of being negative and uncooperative.

Neither Angie nor Erika realize that Martha is keeping their dispute going. Both of them continue in this pattern until 2 weeks later, when Martha is away on vacation. Angie and Erika both notice that shift report seems to go more smoothly but can't figure out why.

Expert Commentary: Vignette 9.4

Competition between colleagues can lead to sabotage and exact a toll on patient care. Sabotaging is a form of lateral violence that needs to be put to a stop as soon as possible. Martha epitomizes the old adage "The dog who carries a bone brings a bone," as she is the bearer of gossip and hurt feelings that keep the feud going.

Angie, Erika, and Martha all play a role in this feud. Talking with them individually and then putting them all in the same room to discuss Angie's and Erika's discovery is the healthiest approach to this triangulated situation. Martha owes them both an apology at a minimum. Other apologies may be in order, depending on other exchanges between Angie and Erika. Martha needs counseling and education on bullying behavior in the workplace. In addition, it would be important to document in her work file.

–G. Rumay Alexander

Angie and Erika, unknown to each of them, are both the victims of bullying behaviors by Martha. Martha utilizes her unique position as intermediary to disrupt the working relationship between Erika and Angie. This is done by gossip and spreading rumors about Erika and Angie to each about the other. The nurse manager may initially view this as a personality clash between Erika and Angie. The improved relationship between these evening and night nurses in the absence of Martha's intermediary role, however, provides the data the nurse manager needs to address the cause of the perceived personality clash. Skillful intervention by the nurse manager will assist Erika and Angie in understanding the root cause of the tension that exists in their working relationship. The nurse manager is in the position to coach Erika and Angie on how they should confront Martha about her bullying behavior and their resolve to stop this directed insidious behavior. It is also likely that similar situations are occurring in the unit. Poor working relationships among and between staff may have its root cause in this bullying behavior.

–M.T. Meadows

This vignette illustrates what can happen when people are not able to debrief following a mistake. The feud between Angie and Erika might actually have been avoided if they both had the opportunity to reflect and comment about the mistake and its contributing factors, instead of Erika stewing over the fact that she had been wrongly accused of an error. Managers can therefore ensure that employees are given an opportunity to debrief following a mistake.

The second issue in this vignette pertains to the fact that both Angie and Erika choose to believe Martha instead of going to each other to validate what was reported about them. Angie is taking Martha's comments at face value, and both Angie and Erika become more and more frustrated as the situation escalates. It is therefore important that employees receive training on how to deal with conflict and to deescalate potentially volatile situations. It is also important that employees be expected to not listen to or take part in gossip. Instead, they can tell the gossiper to stop, that they do not want to hear it. In cases where they feel they have been victimized, employees should confirm with said perpetrator that what they heard is in fact what was said. If the meeting is not successful, they can decide to either speak to their manager or their union representative about the issue.

The last paragraph of this vignette shows Angie and Erika noticing that shift report is smoother since Martha is on vacation, although they are unable to attribute this positive outcome to the role played by Martha in fueling their feud. Because the feud appears to be strictly between Angie and Erika, and because no other peer except for Martha appears to have been privy to the bad feeling between both, it is highly improbable that someone—unless they are made aware of the situation—will be able to help resolve the issue.

One hopes that because the situation between Angie and Erika has somewhat improved, they will be able to openly discuss the issue and conclude that Martha is contributing to their feud by playing both sides against one another, and that they may not actually have said what they were reported to have said. They may then decide to confront Martha about her actions when she returns, or they may choose to tolerate each other while at work without confiding any other information to Martha (refusing to play the game). As a third option, they may decide to inform their unit manager of the issue, so he or she is aware of the fact that Martha's actions may in fact be contributing to conflict and a poor work climate.

–Isabelle St-Pierre

Reflection

Accurate communication between shifts is a patient safety issue. When you audit shift reports, what criteria do you use to determine if vital information is being shared effectively and respectfully? What techniques do you employ if/when you discover that there are deficits in the shift report?

When there are "feuds" between nurses in your unit, at what point do you intervene? What strategies do you use to mediate the conflict?

Vignette 9.5: Super Shift

Jodi, a longtime nurse on the oncology unit at County Hospital, is a friend of Esther, who recently transferred to the ICU. Esther is a bit younger than Jodi and excited by the change in her job.

"You wouldn't believe how good the ICU nurses are!" she says one day, which Jodi takes to mean that the oncology nurses are not good. "We have such great relationships with the docs," Esther says another time. Again, Jodi thinks the relationships with the doctors on the oncology unit are great as well. "You know, you're such a good nurse, you should think about coming to the ICU," Esther suggests. This time, Jodi blows up.

"What do you mean 'such a good nurse'? I love my job just as it is, and being on the oncology floor is my choice!" Thereafter, Jodi hangs out with the ICU clique, and her relationship with Esther is strained.

Expert Commentary: Vignette 9.5

All nurses need to feel a sense of pride in their work and give their best, but there is a thin line between pride and egotism—and that line usually involves status and one-upmanship. It is quite acceptable to challenge one another; however, obsessing on interactions with rivals, comparing notches on the proverbial belt, and overanalyzing rewards and praise can wreak havoc on the bigger goal: good patient care on every floor or unit. Once again, be especially careful with your language. Words create worlds, so their power must be respected. Some feel that certain words, such as "innovation," set people up to play the comparison game, especially if such emotionally laden words are used by the boss. Words can hurt, and words can heal. They can destroy relationships and passion in another for the work that must be performed, or they can assist in the building of generational equity.

Lay the groundwork for reciprocity. Cultivate a spirit of generosity and affirm yourself and others. Spreading negativity throughout the organization is simply not acceptable under any circumstances. To avoid oversights and disruptions, Jodi and Esther would do well to reflect on the lack of professionalism they are modeling for others and the potential danger zone they are creating together, even though that is not their intent. Figuring out ways to affirm each other publicly and privately, share resources, learn from each other, and create collaborative, healthy competitive efforts, such as collecting food for the needy, would be great. It would take the emphasis off self and place it on others.

–G. Rumay Alexander

There appears to be more than one explanation for the resulting loss of friendship between Esther and Jodi. Once again, it is important to determine the cause of the ending of this friendship. Possible explanations include Esther's enthusiasm for her new position in the ICU, generational differences, and Esther's intentional attempts to belittle the oncology unit or place the ICU in higher esteem. In this particular situation, it is important for the nurse managers from both units to be involved in the assessment of the situation.

The ICU nurse manager may discover that a culture of superiority does exist within his or her unit, and that Esther has been quickly socialized into this way of thinking and interacting with peers from other units. The oncology unit nurse manager may discover that generational differences exist in relationship to loyalty to the oncology unit. Jodi values loyalty and may be interpreting Esther's comments as disloyal. Esther, as a younger nurse, has less loyalty to the unit and more toward her peers. Regardless of the reason for the strained relationship between Esther and Jodi, it is important to address and mitigate the cause to ensure a professional working relationship between units, resulting in improved communication and care coordination.

–M.T. Meadows

This last vignette depicts a situation that can in fact be a simple misinterpretation of intent. Esther is excited about her new job and freely shares her feelings and perceptions with Jodi. While Esther never actually compares the ICU nurses to the oncology nurses, Jodi interprets Esther's comments as meaning that she thinks ICU nurses are better. Jodi feels insecure and threatened by Esther's remarks, but instead of validating her perceptions, she lets her emotions escalate out of control and finally lashes out, resulting in Esther withdrawing from the friendship. Once more, this vignette shows the importance of taking the time to validate perceptions before drawing conclusions. If Jodi would have taken the time to verbalize her discomfort and confirm her perceptions with Esther, Esther might have felt bad that her comments were interpreted that way and might have reassured Jodi right away that her intent was not to discredit the oncology nurses.

–Isabelle St-Pierre

Reflection

Nurse managers may also feel that they are in a more prestigious position than the people they supervise. How do you monitor the messages you may consciously or unconsciously give to others about your position within the organization?

How can you and your peer nurse managers promote a sense of pride in the work product of every nurse within your organization?

Summary

When "rankism" occurs at any level, the issues run deeper than the behaviors you observe. A long history of viewing some nurses as "better than" others by virtue of seniority, specialty, or education can create a culture of competition rather than cooperation. While the conflict often plays out on an interpersonal level, everyone within the organization can be affected by it.

As a nurse manager, you may inadvertently buy into a culture of competition. Either you believe your unit is more special than others, or you may feel victimized by your peers, who believe *their* work is the most important and prestigious in the hospital. To begin changing these interactions, activities that focus on commonalities rather than differences can unite rather than divide.

Activities

Encourage your staff (and yourself) to be better at humor than your coworkers. Establish a joke board using a small whiteboard in a prominent place such as the lunchroom, lounge, or locker room. Challenge nurses on each shift to start the next shift's time off with a smile by posting a joke and signing their name. Have the incoming shift award a "smile factor" to the jokes. At the end of the month, give a silly award to the person with the highest smile factor and take him or her out to lunch.

Alternatively, volunteer to facilitate a team-building activity that could be used with either nurses on your unit or your fellow nurse managers. You will need a whiteboard or poster paper.

Make a detailed list of all the things in common among nurses on your unit, such as all of them work in the same physical location, have the same licensure, provide the majority of patient care, are predominantly female, etc. Next, create a list of those things that differ among nurses in the same way. Compare and contrast the two lists, and ask the group to describe how each item on either list impacts patient care.

10 | generations at work

A generation of people consists of the entire body of individuals born and living at about the same time and influenced by the same societal conditions. Sparks (2012) notes four generations of nurses in the workforce: the silent/traditionalist generation (born between 1925 and 1945), baby boomers (born between 1946 and 1964), generation X (born between 1963 and 1980), and millennials (born between 1981 and 2000.

Examining the similarities and differences between these generations can help shed light on some of the intergenerational issues that can arise in the workplace.

- **Silent/traditionalist:** The silent/traditionalist generation (also known as the greatest generation or matures) was raised with strict discipline. Perhaps because of that, members of this generation developed a very hands-off style of child-rearing. As adults, they experienced a boom in divorce rates, placed a high level of importance on wealth, and were very devoted to their job and their work organization. Their pop culture/political reference points are Shirley Temple, Bill Cosby, and Martin Luther King, Jr. (Kauffman, 2012).

- **Baby boomers:** Baby boomers are characterized by their optimistic and generous nature, but also by their rebellious, permissive, and ambitious side. They tend to be deeply invested in their jobs and value hard work. They experienced civil rights, birth control, women's liberation, the moon landing, and the Vietnam and cold wars. Their pop culture/political reference points are Oprah Winfrey, Rush Limbaugh, Hilary Clinton, and Bill Gates (Kauffman, 2012).

- **Generation X:** Generation Xers tend to be fun-loving and self-reliant and value diversity and balance (they work to live, not live to work). They were largely under-protected by their parents and experienced working/single parents, being latchkey children, the space shuttle, the Challenger disaster, Chernobyl, and Watergate. Their pop culture/political reference points are Michael Jordan, Cindy Crawford, Tom Cruise, and Jesse Jackson (Kauffman, 2012).

- **Millennials/Generation Y:** Millennials, who are just entering the workforce, tend to be family oriented, mobile, hopeful, and idealistic. They were raised by "helicopter parents." Millennials tend to value tolerance, cooperation, connection, and novelty. They experienced AIDS, 9/11, global news, climate change, and the Columbine High School massacre. Their pop culture/political reference points are connectedness via technology, Dolly the Sheep, the death of Princess Diana, Bill Clinton, and the television show *Friends* (Kauffman, 2012).

Generation X and baby boomers are two of the largest groups in the workforce today. Yet, these two groups come from very different lived experiences (Kauffman, 2012). According to Amy Sparks (2012), in the workplace, what nurses perceive and value about their working environment differs between generations. Generational differences have been found in many areas, including overall job satisfaction, intent to leave, burnout, work-life balance, and scheduling. There are also generational differences in terms of perception of personal responsibility, autonomy, professional status, and support from leadership (Sparks, 2012).

Working environments that combine these generations—as most do—can be challenging. Differences between generations can become most apparent when working with technology. Mastering technological innovations may flummox some nurses, while others sail right through. For those for whom technology comes easily, it may seem that those who are slower to catch on are stupid or unmotivated. Such intergenerational discord over the technology divide can be disruptive to workplace culture and morale.

Another challenge that arises in an intergenerational workplace is the clash between old and new. Seasoned nurses bring wisdom and experience, and new nurses bring their fresh eyes and recent education. It is a normal, human reaction to highly value that which we personally possess, so new nurses may be more apt to place high value on their education, whereas seasoned nurses may be apt to place a high value on their experience. This can lead to a clash in the workplace, where a new nurse might say, "I learned in school that we should do this procedure X way," and the seasoned nurse replies, "Well, that's not how we do it here."

Managing a multigenerational workforce can be challenging. Sparks proposes the following ideas for coping with intergenerational discord at work:

- Consider the differences between generations, especially with respect to their approach to work and their perspective about work-life balance.

- Talk to individual nurses to gain greater insight into generational trends.

- Hold discussion sessions during annual staff nurse evaluations that enable nurses to discuss their perceptions of their work environment, and remember to think and talk about that information from the perspective of generation (Sparks, 2012).

Vignettes, Commentaries, and Reflective Thinking

The remainder of this chapter presents vignettes about generations at work, commentaries about the experiences represented in the vignettes, and opportunities to explore or reflect on the material.

Vignette 10.1: High Tech

St. Andrews Hospital implements a new "paperless" charting system that requires each unit to gradually transition to electronic charting. On the same-day surgery unit, some nurses are more adept at figuring out the new system and quickly become proficient at using it.

Jami, an older, second-career nurse, worked with technology previously. When Katherine, one of the younger nurses, can't figure out the new system, she offers to help her. "Are you kidding?" says Katherine, who just graduated from her BSN program. "This system is the problem, not me. I've been trying to enter this order for the last 10 minutes, and the screen is frozen."

Jami looks at the screen and presses a refresh button. Quickly, the problem is solved. Katherine glares at her. "I'm sure that would have happened anyway," she says. "I know how to use technology. I did my clinicals in other hospitals where they had a system that worked better."

Katherine continues to have challenges with the system, and each time Jami offers to help, she refuses.

Expert Commentary: Vignette 10.1

Technology innovations can cause a great deal of anxiety for nurses at all levels, because they can create an obstacle in providing direct patient care. Imagine being new to nursing as you try to learn the unit routine and direct patient care for a specific patient population. Next, imagine struggling with an electronic charting system that holds the information you need in order to move forward with the most basic of care. The combination of these circumstances can be paralyzing.

This vignette presents an interesting twist in generational stereotypes. It reminds us that the younger generation, although very technologically savvy, may also have instances when technology is perplexing and overwhelming. Jami, although an older nurse, is a second-degree graduate with technology experience that transfers to her current RN role. Katherine seems to try to downplay any inadequacy she may have in learning the system with statements suggesting that the system is the problem and not her level of understanding or skill. She may not know that Jami holds years of experience in another field that enabled her to develop these technology skills.

Lack of communication is often at the core of conflict for nurses. In this case, it could be lack of communication of orientation goals and outcomes or lack of achievable time frames to acquire and develop the necessary skills to do the job. Observing Jami's approach to providing instruction would be helpful. Is she encouraging or condescending? Is she approachable or standoffish? Is she tactful in providing critiques of Katherine's performance? How could she better provide feedback?

In addition, what is Katherine's self-assessment of her performance? What is working in her orientation? What is not working? What else is going on in Katherine's world that may affect her time at work? What changes can Katherine identify that would help her progress at this time? Does Katherine respond to everyone this way? Is there a better preceptor choice for Katherine at this time?

As a manager, it is important to regularly meet with the new staff member and preceptor together to create open communication of performance and to discuss goals for orientation. In assigning staff to precept, consider the preceptor's personality and characteristics and those of the new nurse, and try to match them when possible. In the initial introductions, it is often helpful to have both parties share basic information about their work experiences, skills, background, likes, and dislikes so that they come together with some beginning understanding of the other person. This can be a first step in building an effective team.

–Mary Lou Kanaskie

Helpful feedback is the nutrient that develops new nurses into accomplished professionals. Here is a wonderful opportunity for the nurse manager, Jami, and Katherine's preceptor to help Katherine learn to accept that she doesn't know everything, and that exposing your ignorance and making mistakes will not be punished on this unit. The values of the unit must be clear: Staff members support each other and explore opportunities to learn, and blaming versus learning just doesn't work here. It would be helpful to have Katherine work with a variety of experienced nurses, so she can learn that collegial relationships will help her to be a better nurse.

–Karlene Kerfoot

Reflection

At the heart of using technology to record and communicate important information is patient care. If nurses on your unit are uncomfortable with electronic charting, what methods can you use to help them? Could Jami and Katherine, as well as other nurses, be partnered to work together in developing training that would facilitate use of technology?

Most hospitals and health care organizations are moving toward electronic records. As institutions become more and more technology oriented, how can nurse managers work with administration to promote careful implementation of new policies and procedures?

Vignette 10.2: Tradition

The oncology unit has a staff of mostly seasoned nurses who have worked at the Springfield Hospital for their whole career. When Valerie, a recent graduate of a nearby BSN program, is hired, the other nurses are skeptical about her ability to learn the ropes.

One day, Valerie allows a husband to stay with his wife while she, Valerie, performs a minor procedure. When Valerie leaves the room, Sandra, the nurse manager, corners her. "Valerie, we never allow visitors in the room when doing a procedure."

"But he's her husband. He'll have to do the same things for her at home in another day or two," Valerie protests.

Later, another nurse, Emily, sees Valerie preparing a "cocktail" of medicines for her patient as ordered and tells her the procedure she is using is wrong. "We always give one medication first, and then wait a few minutes before giving the others," Emily insists.

"But the doctor ordered a 'cocktail,' and that's what I was taught to give," Valerie objects.

After 3 months, Valerie hands in her resignation.

In her exit interview, she tells Sandra, "I really think you need to only hire older nurses here or find someone with thicker skin than me. I got tired of hearing 'That's the way we've always done it' as rationale for all the things I was supposedly doing wrong. Dr. Morgan asked me to be his office nurse, so he must think I'm competent. At least I'll be on my own there and won't be told I'm making mistakes constantly."

Expert Commentary: Vignette 10.2

This case emphasizes the importance of both giving and receiving feedback in constructive ways that are essential for building healthy work relationships. The manager in this example confronts the new nurse about policy but does not inquire about her assessment of the situation or the steps in decision-making that led her to this action. Valerie had an excellent rationale for taking this action. The manager would have been wise to recognize this and to either thank her for pointing out a needed policy change or explain why the existing policy is necessary (such as infection or patient safety).

Another nurse witnessing Valerie's administration of a medication cocktail could have pointed out the way it is intended to be administered and the rationale for giving one medication at a time. The nurse might say, "It is a common misconception that the cocktail can be mixed together, but evidence shows that each drug should be administered separately. If the patient does not tolerate the cocktail and does not take it all, it is not possible to determine how much of any one drug they received." Adding a comment on what she has done well is very important at this time. It sends the message "I want you to succeed and to be the best nurse that you can be."

When new staff members are struggling with criticism, it is so important for them to ask for feedback. This requires them to initiate the conversation by asking, "Please let me know if I've forgotten anything or did not document correctly." This invites others to provide feedback. In doing so, they are more likely to provide helpful feedback in an honest and caring manner. It also confirms for them that this new nurse is conscientious and cares about his or her own performance. Ultimately, it validates that this is someone that they will be glad to work with on the same team.

–Mary Lou Kanaskie

Ensuring that an oncology unit attends to evidence, leading practices, and the highest level of patient safety practices is the responsibility of the professional nurses, the unit leadership, and the hospital. Valerie was utilizing evidence when she assumed the husband needed to be with his wife. And, she was giving the medications as ordered, while the other nurses on the unit were making a very serious legal error by changing the way the physician ordered the medication. With these two blatant examples of below-standard practice, the nurse manager needs to inform the next person in the chain of command to obtain advice about how to handle these problems. The unanticipated exit of a competent new nurse with only 3 months' tenure is costly and should place the nurse manager on high alert that there are serious quality and potential financial problems on the unit that must be attended to immediately to address the patient safety and legal issues.

How did the unit get to this point, and what needs to be done? There are four main issues to address:

- When cliques form within units and its members isolate themselves from others, the result is a lack of teamwork and of positive valuing of others. The clique sets up informal rules on the unit that allow this behavior to exist. Integration of members of the unit can be accomplished by integrating schedules, committee assignments, etc. When people are less isolated, differences are less noticeable.

- There is a lack of evidence-based practice. Practicing by evidence needs to be implemented.

- The nurse manager needs to take a strong stand against the practices.

- Nursing staff members need to recognize they are not practicing at a professional level and must work with the nurse manager and other superiors to build the infrastructure to handle that. The staff must be involved and held accountable for positive onboarding, retention, and nurse satisfaction; must practice excellence; and must be concerned about unexpected exits of competent nurses.

–Karlene Kerfoot

Reflection

What learning opportunities do you see in the vignette above? If this situation occurred on your unit, what steps would you take to educate all employees on communication and constructive feedback?

New nurses are vulnerable to disappointment and doubt related to their new job. Losing a nurse before orientation is completed is costly to both the organization and you as a manager. How does your unit compare with others on retaining new nurses beyond the orientation period? If there is room for improvement, what ideas do you have about ways to do so?

Vignette 10.3: Allegiance

At State Hospital, there are two cohorts of nurses: those who have worked at the institution for a long time and are location bound, and those who are more mobile and transient. Cara, a longtimer, has seen a parade of new nurses going through the psych unit in recent months and begins to resent those who come and go quickly. "Call me old-fashioned, but there's something to be said for loyalty," she tells Lorraine, a nurse who has been on the psych unit for less than a year.

"But nowadays, people move. If your husband gets a new job, you're likely to have to move to accommodate it," Lorraine replies.

"Maybe, but you can tell these new nurses don't care at all about this unit or the patients here. It's just a job to them." Although Lorraine doesn't argue, she knows that "these new nurses" find Cara difficult to work with because of her attitude toward them.

Expert Commentary: Vignette 10.3

It is difficult for experienced staff to precept new nurses and witness them time and again leaving just as they are becoming productive members of the team. Preceptors expend a tremendous amount of energy and at times, can be emotionally drained. The challenge for the manager is to create a unit culture that celebrates loyalty and the expertise that comes with years of experience while reaching out to new staff members to join the team.

The opportunity to work with and learn from an experienced staff can be a great recruitment tool if the concept is planted and nourished by the manager. In addition, the manager can encourage the staff to embrace the reality that some members of the team will be mobile and that although their time with the team will be short, the team will have prepared them with the knowledge and skills to embark on new nursing adventures. For that, they can be very proud.

–Mary Lou Kanaskie

Diversity is the hallmark of nursing. There is plentiful evidence of the generational differences of nurses and their expectations and values. Successful units honor and value generational differences and celebrate that everyone contributes to the unit in his or her own special way. After providing information to the unit shared governance council about the evidence of generational differences in nursing, and after discussing the staff feedback with Cara, the nurse manager could ask Cara to lead a group discussion about how the unit can be more effective in honoring and accommodating differences on the unit.

–Karlene Kerfoot

Reflection

What are the pros and cons of a "merry-go-round" situation where new nurses come and go, while a stable cohort of employees continues for years and even decades? Might this create an experience gap—where there are lots of nurses with decades of experience and lots of brand-new nurses, but no one with several years experience? Is this a problem? If so, why?

Although some nurses may come to your unit knowing their tenure will be short, what can you and other nurse managers do to promote a sense of loyalty and commitment to the hospital, even if they're only there on a short-term basis?

Vignette 10.4: In for the Long Haul

Rita has been working in the ICU for 10 months in anticipation of going to graduate school and becoming a nurse anesthetist. She is conscientious with her patients and helps out her coworkers as needed, but for the most part, she keeps to herself.

Ruth, who has been at the ICU for 5 years, voices her feelings about Rita at shift change one day. "She's an opportunist. She's just working here so she can get into anesthesia school, and everyone knows it. She could care less about this place."

Marilyn, another more seasoned nurse, joins in. "She has her nose up in the air because she thinks she's better than us."

The evening nurses don't know much about Rita. After hearing Ruth and Marilyn put her down, however, they decide the complaints must be true. They begin scrutinizing Rita's patient care. Thereafter, they manage to find small things to criticize Rita for: supplies that weren't replaced promptly, charting that isn't 100% complete, and a patient who needed pain medication and didn't get it. (The 4-hour "prn" time period hadn't elapsed during Rita's shift, but the evening nurses didn't bother to note that.) The evening nurses make sure to pass on their observations to the nurse manager so Rita can be given their "feedback."

Expert Commentary: Vignette 10.4

As in the previous vignette, it is difficult for experienced staff to precept new nurses only to see them leave their unit after 1 year. This situation is very common in intensive care units (ICUs), where nurses begin their employment to obtain the required experience for nurse anesthetist or nurse practitioner programs, never intending to make ICU nursing their career choice. This is a workplace reality. The challenge for nursing leaders is to welcome these new members of the profession and encourage them on their chosen career paths while building a unit culture that supports this important work and builds the self-esteem of the staff.

The sabotage and bullying seen in this case are congruent with the powerlessness, lack of control, and lack of self-esteem often related to these behaviors. The act of not giving direct feedback but telling others and trying to negatively influence others' beliefs is all too common. Managers can stop this specific behavior by describing it to the offenders and by providing them with help to provide direct peer review. Formal and informal sessions can be conducted to discuss peer-review techniques and the importance of open, honest, and constructive communication to ensure a safe patient-care environment. Practicing the words to use in different situations is very useful as these skills are developed.

–Mary Lou Kanaskie

Unfortunately, there is an element of antiintellectualism among some RNs. For example, nurses who have progressed from an ADN to a BSN may be criticized and labeled "too academic" by those who choose not to pursue educational advancement. Of course the culture of the unit has allowed and reinforced this view when it becomes the prevailing norm of the unit, instead of celebrating educational advancement. Some ICU units become learning laboratories for nurses needing experience to advance toward becoming a specialized nurse practitioner. Instead of being critical of nurses who want to advance making this choice, the unit needs to see that they are very special and can have as their mission supporting people who want to advance.

There also is the "boiled lobster" syndrome in nursing. As lobsters try to crawl out of the pot of boiling water, the lobsters on the bottom pull them back into the lethal waters. Rather than celebrating others' success, we too often find people criticizing others and trying to pull them back down with criticism. Cultures that celebrate success will "do no harm" to others.

Culture is nothing more than a summary of behaviors that are and are not allowed. Strong nurse leaders create positive or negative cultures. These leaders can be staff nurses, managers, and organizational leaders who create the culture. We can proactively create cultures in which patients and staff are cared for and cared about and where there is zero tolerance for nurses who hurt other nurses.

The rules of a culture can be formally described and taught. Alternatively, they can be the informal rules that are not directly expressed but subtly taught by positive or negative feedback. In high-performing organizations, clear mission statements and values become an integral part of the organization and unit, rather than merely hanging on the wall and not becoming integrated within the culture.

Leaders need objective data about the health of the culture, gleaned through the use of focus groups, formal employee surveys, and specialized surveys tailored to RNs. Just as we do root-cause analysis for sentinel events when patient care goes wrong, a root-cause analysis of dysfunctional events will uncover defects in the health of the unit. In this situation, it is apparent that generational differences and separation of nurses into cliques were at least some of the causes of the dysfunctional behavior. It may be that the values of the organization are not a part of the everyday workings on the unit. This would indicate to the nurse manager and staff that it's necessary to reteach these values. Inadequate enforcement for breaches of values by the nurse manager and the professional peer-review process could also be problems. Changing the assignments to ensure that staff members have the opportunity to work with a variety of people instead of their clique could be another option to avoid isolating into dysfunctional groups. Just as collegial, intraprofessional groups create the best outcomes, so do integrated, respectful groups of intergenerational nurses working collaboratively in teams.

–Karlene Kerfoot

Reflection

What alternative learning opportunities can be offered to nurses who may not be able to engage in formal continuing education?

How can you recognize the accomplishments of all nurses without creating an environment of negative competition?

Summary

As hospitals employ a greater mix of nurses at different stages and ages of their professional careers, these differences can create tensions. Being explicit about how loyalty and work ethic plays out on your unit can help employees see that there is no single "correct" attitude. As a nurse manager, it is your job to stress that the "glue" of quality patient care holds all members of the team together, regardless of their work status.

At the same time, a big part of teamwork is recognizing and appreciating differences. Being able to promote friendly dialogue about generational values can defuse tension and promote bonding. We all like to learn about ourselves and the people we work with—so encourage sharing! As nurses' communication and connection skills improve, their ability to give and receive helpful feedback will follow.

Activity

Have a day when everyone brings in a picture of themselves in nursing school or at a younger age. (Doing this during Nurses Week works well.) Display the photos on a wall to see if individuals can be identified from the images. Ask each nurse to describe the process they learned for giving medications as a student or to share a "new practice" they learned while they were being trained. For example, when many older nurses went to nursing school, repair of an inguinal hernia was done on an inpatient basis, and patients were expected to stay in bed for several days postop. Now it's outpatient therapy!

Sharing stories can help nurses appreciate perspectives and promote understanding. If you want to be really ambitious, pull a headline or newspaper clip-out from the year each nurse graduated to facilitate further dialogue.

---

11 | minimizing the value of colleagues

According to our review, nurse managers and administrators are often thought to be less clinically competent than the nurses they supervise. In particular, staff nurses said that being promoted to a position of nurse manager or administrator did not necessarily signify better nursing skills, earn greater respect, or improve relationships.

A belief that management is somehow separate or different from front-line nurses makes it difficult for both groups to collaborate, respect each other, or work as a team. Some nurses feel nurse managers and administrators have lost touch with the realities of clinical nursing and go out of their way to avoid becoming involved in activities at the bedside, even when their efforts are clearly needed. At the same time, nurse managers as well as front-line nurses can be frustrated by nurses who create "drama" and seem to be self-centered and uninterested in teamwork.

Commentator Melissa Snyder highlights the relational component to minimizing the value of colleagues. She notes the following:

> *Although everyone is faced with busy schedules and demanding roles, the relationship piece cannot be overlooked. In order to build effective professional relationships, nurse managers must provide frequent opportunities for staff to share their concerns and suggestions for improvements; managers must act on these discussions and demonstrate an interest in supporting staff nurses in all aspects of their*

roles. Taking opportunities several times a week to visit the staff nurses in their environment can be very effective, especially if there is no purpose other than to see how things are going. Additionally, when the nurse manager is contacted for help with difficult situations, the nurse manager ought to provide consistent support until the problem is solved. This support can be conveyed by maintaining frequent contact, creating a clearly defined plan or timeline for how the problem will be resolved, and following up with contacts until resolution of the problem is achieved. Staff nurses want their nurse managers to be resources and advocates for their needs.

Gardner (2005) writes about the importance of collaboration in all disciplines but emphasizes that in health care, this behavior can improve patient outcomes, increase nursing satisfaction, and improve teamwork. She offers 10 excellent tips, summarized below, which are useful for both managers and team members:

- Know thyself. Understand how your own values, assumptions, and expectations shape behavior. Effective collaboration and teamwork in the health care environment require constant reevaluation and resetting. Each worker must set aside personal feelings and concentrate on the common goal of patient care.

- Learn to value and manage diversity, even though nursing remains a relatively nondiverse profession, at least in terms of gender. Appreciating the difference in communication styles between men and women and physicians and nurses as well as those from other cultures can help nurses be cognitively diverse. Cognitive diversity expands the resources available for collaboration in any given situation.

- Use constructive conflict-management skills that enhance collaboration. Accepting the existence of conflict and opening a constructive dialogue is more productive than avoiding or denying conflict.

- Identify win-win situations that reflect compromise and the value of the team collaboration over individual power. Even if you believe you are right, the choice of behavior and actions should be determined by consensus of team members and directed toward the best possible patient care.

- Develop effective interpersonal skills. Although nurses are often very good at communicating and relating to patients, they may be less invested in using the same behaviors with coworkers. Team members must be comfortable with themselves and have confidence in not only their own abilities but in those of their colleagues. Conflict often arises when one nurse feels threatened, envious, or resentful of another.

- View teamwork as a journey, not a destination. Relationships and collaboration need to be reevaluated and renewed constantly as the environment changes. The process of reconnecting around patient needs is never static.

- Share decision-making to increase collaboration. Joint clinical rounds and interdisciplinary team meetings provide an opportunity to make connections and ground relationships before a crisis occurs.

- Allow teams to occur spontaneously and without scripting. If two or three nurses have a special interest in pursuing a particular subject or issue, allow it to happen organically, rather than trying to micromanage or join in.

- Understand that teams involve both autonomy and unity. Gardner (2005) warns against static patterns of interaction. Rather, a blend of both individual interests and group dynamics can maximize teamwork and collaboration.

- Not every decision requires collaboration and teamwork. Sometimes, decisions need to be made unilaterally, but complex problems usually benefit from collaborative problem-solving.

Kalish, Lee, and Rochman (2010) studied a sample of 3,675 nurses to determine the impact of nursing teams. Not surprisingly, a higher degree of teamwork led to a higher degree of job satisfaction and other variables connected to it. When nurses feel connected, appreciated, and empowered, they are willing to work under less-than-ideal circumstances. All these conditions are affected by the nurse manager, who must interface both with management to mobilize people and resources and with leadership to provide influence and vision—all the while addressing role stressors and challenges (Zastocki & Holly, 2010).

Wilson et al. (2005) reviewed the literature and found that communication needed to be of the closed-loop variety, meaning that everyone knew the same information. They also concluded that collaboration offsets error. Coworkers need to ask for help when they need it, be aware of the needs of their coworkers, and offer help freely. Deference to expertise was also important, but expertise was not necessarily due to the person's status within the institution. A collective orientation leads to the belief that the actions of each individual affects the whole team.

Barrett, Korber, Padula, and Piatek (2009) found that an intervention designed to build a sense of teamwork was greatly negatively affected by high turnover among nurse managers as well as the status of nurse managers who were in a place of crisis during the study. Ironically, the individual most responsible for the function of the team (the nurse manager) was least available to help.

Unfortunately, turnover among nurse managers, which can be as rapid as turnover among nurses, can cause a team to fall apart. Zastocki and Holly (2010) note the crucial role of the nurse manager in every organization, registering concern over the shrinking number of qualified nurse managers. They report that in some places, there is an 8.3% vacancy rate among nurse managers.

Shared decision-making also contributes to satisfaction and helps nurses feel in charge of their workplace. In a study of more than 3,000 nurses from 80 patient-care units, Kalish, Lee, and Rochman (2010) discovered that the Nursing Teamwork Survey connected a number of variables and positive outcomes to the individual nurse's sense of perceived teamwork and collaboration.

While it used to be standard practice for the nurse manager to be autocratic, Wilson et al. (2005) believe that shared decision-making is now essential—not as an occasional gesture but as an ongoing practice the manager believes is best. They encourage nurse managers to engage staff in project teams, provide clear directions, and participate in their meetings.

Wilson found that conflict occurred not because of hierarchy or power struggles, but because team cohesiveness got blocked. In a similar study, nurses connected relationships with their nurse manager and workplace conflict (Almost Doran, McGillis Hall, & Spence Laschinger, 2010). Learning to manage conflict might not prevent conflict, but some of the negative consequences could be mediated.

Spence Laschinger (2010) points out that nurses constitute the largest group of professionals in the health care environment. As such, they are the most at-risk for stress and burnout. The mediating variable in this situation is relationships with coworkers, which nurses commented on again and again. Where a sense of cooperation and collaboration prevailed, nurses were resilient in the face of a variety of workplace challenges. Spence Laschinger (2010) expresses the possibility that nurse managers can help shape a positive, respectful working environment. Still, each nurse must take accountability for giving respect to and receiving respect from all coworkers at a minimum.

Vignettes, Commentaries, and Reflective Thinking

The remainder of this chapter presents vignettes about minimizing the value of colleagues, commentaries about the experiences represented in the vignettes, and opportunities to explore or reflect on the material.

Vignette 11.1: Those Who Can

Hannah is frustrated by her clinical head nurse, Jessica. Last week, Hannah was working with a patient who has a ventricular assist device (VAD) that didn't seem to want to cooperate. Hannah asked Jessica for help troubleshooting the problem, so Jessica came in and took a look. After trying unsuccessfully to help, Jessica said, "Well the patient looks fine," and left!

Hannah vents to a coworker about how this type of thing happens frequently: Someone asks a clinical head for help, but then the clinical head isn't able to help. Hannah says, "I just feel like I can't count on Jessica to help when I need actual clinical input. She's good at being an advocate for nurses, but not at the bedside stuff. I can't imagine being her patient, and that really decreases my confidence in her. And I feel about half the leadership in our unit is like this—I just don't trust their clinical judgment, which makes it really hard to respect them as leaders of a clinical unit!"

Expert Commentary: Vignette 11.1

Hannah appropriately seeks advice and guidance from her clinical head nurse, Jessica, regarding a specific, technical patient-care issue. It is reasonable for Hannah to expect that she will receive some degree of assistance with the VAD that is causing trouble for both her and her patient. In the past, Hannah has been disappointed with the clinical head nurse's input regarding clinical challenges. She is again disappointed. Jessica doesn't know the answer, can't fix the problem, and offers no alternative solutions. In frustration, Hannah admits that she loses respect and confidence in Jessica as a clinical leader when these things happen.

Medical devices can pose problems for anyone from time to time. Because Jessica has different responsibilities on the unit than the bedside nurse, she may not have as much experience with troubleshooting VAD technical problems. However, Jessica needs to know where to find the answers. A leader doesn't need to know all of the answers all of the time. A leader needs to know whom to call and where to look to find the answers. Instead of dismissing Hannah's dilemma and walking away, Jessica could have offered other helpful resources: Check the policy, consult the VAD manual, contact the device representative using the 1-800 number printed on the equipment, access the manufacturer's website, or page the hospital's VAD program coordinator. Knowing these resources and helping Hannah find the answer to this patient-care problem would generate respect and trust in Jessica's leadership abilities. Working together to find the answers provides Jessica an opportunity to coach Hannah and arm her with resources to use in future situations.

–Carol Tringali

Clinical competence is important for all nurses working in a clinical setting. It is important to clearly delineate the roles and expectations of all levels of nursing, from the nurse manager to the nurse educator to the direct-care nurses. Hannah's comments indicate a few things.

First, Hannah seems to express concern that she is not being supported by the individuals she perceives to be the experts on the unit. This concern may be rooted in fear that if something does go wrong, who will be there to help her and her patient? It would be helpful for the nurse manager to address these concerns directly with Hannah. Is there some type of education or other resources that would help build Hannah's confidence in her own abilities? Is there a more-experienced nurse who could mentor Hannah? It may also be that Hannah does not clearly understand the role of a nurse manager or clinical head nurse on this unit, and her expectations for this role are not aligned with the actual position description. This issue needs to be discussed.

Secondly, the nurse manager's response when Hannah seeks her assistance is not very helpful. If the nurse manager is unable to solve a problem directly, it is imperative that she not leave the situation until the needed assessment and resources have been provided. The staff nurse is simply looking for support and help with problem-solving. If the nurse manager does not provide this, she has failed to gain the trust and respect of the staff nurse. Staff nurses generally do not expect the nurse manager to know the solution for every problem, but they do expect the nurse manager to help identify solutions to their problems.

Finally, it is important that recognition is provided for all roles on a particular unit. Clearly defined position descriptions will set the foundation, but routinely, the staff needs to be reminded of the positive contributions every member is making to the success of the unit. Identifying these contributions helps staff members respect and value the roles of all colleagues.

–Melissa Snyder

Reflection

How do you help the nurses on your unit understand the roles and responsibilities of the various colleagues they may encounter during their work time?

What can nurse managers such as you do to maintain clinical competence, or do you feel this isn't necessary at your institution?

When equipment fails, what resources are available for your nurses, especially during shifts and weekends when regular staff may not be available?

Vignette 11.2: Back in the Day

June works on a med-surg acute care floor. She is taking care of a patient who tells her he plans to attempt suicide. June tells Grace, her manager, about the patient's statement. Grace reminds June about the hospital policy on suicide precautions, which includes a 1:1 ratio and stripping the room of any potentially dangerous items. Two hours later, June is still waiting for an aide to show up to serve as the 1:1 for her patient. Grace says, "Sorry, there's no 1:1 available right now. Just do your best."

June is frustrated and vents to her friend Allison. "Grace has completely forgotten what it's like to be at the bedside! I have this patient, along with my four other patients, and of course because he's on suicide precaution, he's a ton of extra work. I mean, this patient *per hospital policy* is a lot of work, and Grace is just totally unhelpful!"

Allison commiserates. "I know what you mean. If Grace had any memory of what it was like to care for four patients—let alone a patient on suicide precaution—she would never leave you stranded like that to fend for yourself!"

Expert Commentary: Vignette 11.2

When a person expresses thoughts of suicide, the statement must be taken seriously, and further assessment is immediately required to determine patient risk factors and overt suicidal ideation. If the patient states that he or she is currently suicidal, is able to outline a suicide plan, is noted to have poor impulse control, or is found to have multiple risk factors for suicide, then 24-hour observation is required to maintain patient safety.

June is correct to report to her manager the patient's statement about having plans to attempt suicide. Grace has the patient's safety in mind when she reminds June of the policy to remove potentially dangerous materials from the patient's room and provide 1:1 observation. However, neither June nor Grace has indicated whether a suicide risk assessment was completed to determine whether this patient is at immediate risk (requiring immediate 1:1) or is not presently suicidal and, therefore, requires merely frequent observation and prompt evaluation by the psychiatric consult service. The risk assessment must be conducted immediately and documented. Most hospital policies state that a 1:1 ratio of continuous observation for immediate-risk patients can be initiated by the nurse in the interest of patient safety but must be ordered by the physician within a certain time frame. The 1:1 is then to be managed by trained staff, and at no time can the patient be left alone. If June is obliged to provide 1:1 care for this patient, she cannot be expected to also care for her other assigned patients.

June feels abandoned because of the nurse manager's lack of support and leadership in this difficult and stressful situation. Although Grace attempted to find coverage for the 1:1, 2 hours have elapsed without a backup plan or reassignment of responsibilities. This puts the suicidal patient at risk as well as June's other patients. It has also caused June additional stress as she tries to provide safe care to all five of her patients. Even as Grace was trying to get help, contingency plans needed to be developed. Responsibility for this patient could be shared among all the nurses on duty, each taking a turn providing one hour of 1:1 observation, while the other nurses covered their assignments. Alternatively, June's patients could be reassigned so she can supervise the suicidal patient. When June discussed the problem with Allison, the two of them could have developed a plan of mutual support to get the patient care done.

Patient safety is a priority. As the nurse manager, Grace is responsible for the safety of all the patients on her unit and for providing a healthy work environment for her staff. Suicide is a preventable death that is devastating for the family and the nursing staff. Accurate assessment and ongoing communication foster the teamwork necessary to provide care that is in the best interest of the patient.

–Carol Tringali

In this scenario, patient safety is central. The nurse manager is recognizing the safety risk but is not actively pursuing a solution to the problem beyond requesting an aide, who is unavailable at that time. The frustration of June and Allison is that the nurse manager is not doing "enough" to support them in their demanding positions.

A better approach by the nurse manager would have been to relay the message about the delay in getting an aide but to then help June develop a plan for how to meet her patients' needs during the interim. This could be as simple as asking another nurse to provide support for one or two of June's other patients or taking some of her own time to sit with the suicidal patient while June provided care to her other patients. The nurse manager can convey her concern by returning to check on progress with the situation within a short period of time. Most importantly, the nurse manager must demonstrate that she is advocating for June and the other nurses on the unit by addressing their needs with higher levels of administration. The staff nurses must be given opportunities to ask questions and vent their frustrations about their jobs directly to the nurse manager. These venting sessions could result in a list of concerns and suggestions for improvements that address the staff nurses' needs.

–Melissa Snyder

Reflection

Both staff and management can be caught "between a rock and a hard place" due to hospital policies. How do you work with your employees to come up with a mutually satisfactory solution to the problem when such situations occur?

When hospital policies that impact most directly on your staff cause difficulty, how do you follow up with both other nurse managers and higher administration?

Do your nurses respect your clinical acumen? Do you show them that you remember what their job is like and that you respect and appreciate the work they do? If not, how can you work to make these changes?

What data do you collect when situations such as the one above occur? If/when you approach administration, how do you go about requesting a reexamination of the policy?

Vignette 11.3: Spotty Management

Many of the nurses at St. Francis East Hospital feel like their nurse managers no longer make regular rounds, relying on unit managers to keep them informed. The feeling among staff is that the nurse managers in general have no idea what's really going on in their units.

One day, a crisis breaks out in the medical IMCU. Immediately following two new admissions, two patients go into cardiac arrest almost simultaneously. Elaine, the charge nurse on the unit, does her best to help keep things organized, but at a certain point, she really needs the help of her nurse manager, Connie. Connie arrives on the unit in response to the cardiac arrest, gets a quick report from the unit secretary, and then exits.

"Figures," Elaine says. "No one is ever around to help when you need it. They have no idea what goes on out here."

A few minutes later, Ruby, an LPN who floats throughout the hospital, reports in to Elaine.

"Connie told me there were some things going on that you could use help with," she says. "You're lucky she's got your back. Other supervisors never even leave their office."

Elaine accepts the help and the information but thinks to herself, "This isn't my job! I need leadership support. I need Connie to be around more often."

Expert Commentary: Vignette 11.3

Communication is a vital element of all interpersonal interactions. In times of crisis, it becomes more crucial. For people who have developed trust and confidence in each other based on experience working closely together toward mutual goals, words don't always have to be spoken to accomplish effective communication. Eye contact, a gesture, or a nonverbal signal can indicate support or understanding of what is needed. However, clarifying the message is also an important piece of effective communication, because what one sees or hears may be perceived inaccurately.

Connie, the nurse manager, made an assessment of the situation on the unit from visual clues and a report from the secretary. She did not speak to Elaine, nor was there any nonverbal interaction between the two before Elaine saw Connie leave the floor. Perhaps Connie thought Elaine was too busy to be approached. Connie rightly assessed that additional help was needed, but she assumed that another nurse would fill the need. However, if she had asked Elaine, "How can I help? Let me see if I can float someone up here," Elaine might have identified some other immediate needs—someone to provide emotional support to the families of the critical patients, someone to check on the newly admitted patients to inquire about unmet needs, or someone to touch base with her staff nurses to help them get back on track after the cardiac arrests. Elaine, herself, may have needed a supportive person to listen to her recount the events that just happened and confirm everything was handled correctly. Rather than exit the unit abruptly, Connie's presence to help organize and guide would demonstrate the support and teamwork of leadership.

It's a plus that Ruby can voice her positive thoughts about Connie as a nurse manager who cares about her staff. Ruby's remarks have healing power and may serve to give Elaine the confidence to discuss her feelings about this situation with Connie. The relationship between Connie and Elaine needs to be built on trust and an understanding of the expectations each one has of the other.

Nurse leaders who practice transformational leadership delicately balance openness with direction and discipline toward adherence to standards of performance. They recognize the value of engagement with their staff. Rather than dictate, transformational leaders mentor their nurses, challenge them to share creative ideas, and motivate them to produce innovative strategies to solve problems. The self-esteem generated through use of these leadership principles cultivates collaboration between staff and their nurse manager or clinical head nurse, empowers staff to speak up respectfully about needs and expectations, and fosters teamwork.

–Carol Tringali

This scenario points to the importance of the nurse manager being "present" to the staff. Although demands on the nurse manager's time are significant, this is never an excuse for not being available to staff members who require your attention and support. Making a point of getting to know staff members and routinely visiting their workspace send the message that the nurse manager is interested in their needs and aware of the activities in their unit.

When problems develop, the staff will be more likely to seek the guidance of the nurse manager who has a vested interest in their work and will feel confident that their needs will be responded to in an appropriate way. Connie's actions as the nurse manager do not convey any type of relationship to the staff or interest in the outcomes of the situation. It would have been appropriate for Connie to speak directly to Elaine and to reassure her that she would be sending appropriate staff support. Instead, Elaine felt abandoned at a critical time.

From Elaine's perspective, it would be important to share her concerns and frustrations with her nurse manager and to seek a more effective relationship. As the charge nurse, Elaine is in a position to directly address this issue and to request more direct interaction with management. Ultimately, staff satisfaction and patient outcomes will be directly influenced by the relationships that are established between staff nurses and nurse managers.

–Melissa Snyder

Reflection

What strategies do you use to monitor the "emotional temperature" of your unit? Can you tell when nurses are in over their heads and need your assistance, or do you wait for them to come to you with requests for help?

Crises require a special kind of management skill. What behaviors do you pull into play when there is a crisis on your unit and everyone is looking to you for leadership?

Knowing when—and how—to ask for help is a critical skill for any manager. When do you turn to your supervisor or administrator for help?

Summary

Respect for and confidence in coworkers are essential on health care teams, yet often, little time is spent on the "people skills" that make collaboration effective. Your staff may not appreciate the competing tensions you, as nurse manager, face as the go-between. On one side is administration, pressuring you to meet metrics and monitor productivity, while on the other side are those who work for you, hoping that you will provide them with support, understanding, and clinical expertise.

This is when your peer nurse managers can form a support group that can help you make your way through the maze of management. While we often assign preceptors to new nurses, doing the same for new nurse managers is practically unheard of!

At the same time, you need to know your staff and be as transparent with them as you expect them to be with you. Don't wait until performance reviews to discuss strengths and weaknesses—touch base often with those who work for you, asking them to identify areas where they think the team could be strengthened. Share your own perceptions, too.

Make sure to let everyone know when things go well, too. It's fine to process and deconstruct critical incidents or other events where a breakdown in care occurs, but it's also important to recognize when things went well. Take the opportunity to acknowledge excellent teamwork, and you'll give your staff an example of behaviors they should strive for on a daily basis!

Activities

Establish a "Colleague Recognition Day." For each employee on your unit, create an index card that says, "I appreciate you because:_____." You can start with a particular color of card for nurses and then work through support staff and others with a different color of card. Put one nurse's name on the top of each card.

(continues)

(continued)

Then give every nurse an index card with the name of another nurse and instructions to complete it and give it to the person whose name they drew. The idea is that each nurse gets one and each nurse gives one. Depending on your staff, you may want to prep them with some guidance about appreciating each person's contribution at work and recognizing that everyone contributes something.

Alternatively, post a large piece of paper in, say, the locker room and title it "Random Acts of Kindness." Provide sticky notes and ask employees to write something encouraging or positive that a coworker did and post it on the paper. The "poster" can be anonymous, but the "postee" (the person who performed the random act of kindness) should be identified. The nurse manager can also post to level the playing field.

Or, implement weekly "debriefing" sessions. You might use a whiteboard and post it in the lounge, or poll different employees each week. Use a "Roses and Thorns" type activity where nurses can write (or submit anonymous comments to you) on something positive that happened in the last week and an area that could be strengthened. Although the list will change from week to week, you can keep track of themes in the feedback you get and create an action plan to address specific areas that need attention.

part IV sinister systems

12 | politics and CYA

A friend of ours is a nurse—let's call her "April." After getting her nursing degree, April almost immediately became a stay-at-home mom. It was only within the last few years that she has gotten back into the workforce. April's an excellent nurse. She enjoys the work of nursing, but the thing she likes best is really the people. April's baseline *modus operandi* is silliness. She constantly jokes with the patients and their families, telling stupid knock-knock jokes and self-deprecating one-liners. The patients love April. April loves the patients. So everything's good, right?

Unfortunately, no. April is seriously considering looking for a new job, despite the fact that she's only been in her present position for a little over a year. The reason she's unhappy at work doesn't have anything to do with the work of being a nurse. It's not the patients. It's not the families. It's the politics. It's the way leadership never asks her input about changes that affect her daily practice. It's the fact that those changes seem to come down from on high, with no discussion or debate—just, "Do this now." It's the heated conflicts between stakeholders that she has to intentionally distance herself from.

Commentator Donna Kandsberger notes the following:

It is often said that "change is the only constant," and this is particularly true in today's health care environment. However, this doesn't make change less stressful or challenging for all of those attempting to deal with it. When work situations are constantly shifting, nurses may fear the outcomes of change, particularly those that could result in the loss of benefits such as job security, preferred work schedule, or other conditions that make a job person-ally and professionally satisfying. When this happens, the potential benefits the change is intended to create can go unrecognized, more so if it is focused on the macro rath-er than the micro level. Small or large losses of routine, stability, or tangible benefits to some individuals can be threatening, especially when the reason for the change or the intended benefit is not clearly understood by all those who will be affected.

CYA (cover your ass) policies can contribute to office politics and an unhealthy working environment. For example, when a front-line nurse is asked to carry out a plan of care that was developed based on a CYA policy for patient restraints, that nurse is more likely to feel as though her institution is not look-ing out for her, that her managers don't remember what it's like at the bedside, and that she's floating alone in her role with no real support. These feelings can contribute to a trait called orga-nizational cynicism, which is covered in more depth in Chapter 16, "Toxic Culture/Environment."

In a *Wall Street Journal* how-to guide called "How to Han-dle Office Politics," the author begins, "Some people steer clear of office politics, but playing the game may be crucial for career success, because it offers a way to learn how power and influ-ence are managed in your company" ("How to Handle Office Politics," 2012, para.1). Although this sentiment strikes us as reflective of a very sad state of affairs, we're not sure the author is entirely wrong. The fact of the matter is that most folks have to deal with office politics to a certain extent, and knowing how to do it well can be a serious advantage.

But what can a manager do to try to minimize the amount of office politics and the potential negative consequences? Here are a few ideas:

- Hire people with the right kind of ambition. This means looking for people whose ambition is the *com-pany's* success, not necessarily their own.

- Build processes for potentially political issues and do not deviate from them. Certain activities tend to promote political behavior:
  - Performance evaluation and compensation
  - Organizational design, territory, and change
  - Promotions

If you handle these types of activities the same way every time, it will reduce the chances that staff members will complain they were treated unfairly or that the organization and leadership do not have their best interests at heart. Unfortunately, though, the bottom line is that it is probably impossible to escape from office politics in nursing. Whether you're a float nurse, a bedside nurse, a nurse leader, or the chief nursing officer, politics will follow you wherever you go. The best—perhaps only—thing you can do is to realize it's inevitable and try to reduce the negative consequences for yourself and others.

Vignettes, Commentaries, and Reflective Thinking

The remainder of this chapter presents vignettes about hospital politics, commentaries about the experiences represented in the vignettes, and opportunities to explore or reflect on the material.

Vignette 12.1: Mergers/Demergers

Biggs Medical Center and Johns Hospital South decide to merge their efforts and provide better care for residents in their catchment area. The nurses in each institution lose seniority as positions are merged and the administrative structure changes. "I wish this whole merger had never happened," Ashley, an LPN, complains to Karen, her manager, one day.

"Be thankful you have a job," Karen advises. "Biggs Medical Center doesn't use LPNs, and for awhile, there was discussion of not having any positions at all after the merger." Stunned,

Ashley keeps her thoughts to herself from that point forward. Some nurses, however, continue to find fault with the new structure and believe that the merger was prompted by money more than the desire to provide better patient care. Other nurses who have been adversely affected by the merger agree but fear to speak up, because their jobs might be endangered.

Expert Commentary: Vignette 12.1

Mergers and demergers are often strategic decisions that cannot be openly discussed and communicated in the early phases until the legal and financial arrangements are known and studied. When people in the organization are surprised by the news, they may feel betrayed because they were not informed at an earlier point in the discussion. The health care systems of today will experience more mergers and demergers as new relationships develop. This is because the reimbursement system is rapidly changing, making it more difficult for standalone, community-based hospitals to remain financially solvent.

A merger with another hospital or health system produces a great deal of anxiety for people in every role within both organizations. Fear is a powerful emotion and may bring out the worst in people. People involved in this level of change are often fearful of the unknown. They really want to know how the change will affect *them*. The challenge for nurse leaders is that they may not have that answer right away. Without factual information, staff will begin to fill in the blanks themselves—even if the information is not truthful. The rumor mill can become very active and will contribute to an environment of fear, as discussed in this vignette.

In a case like this, leadership should be truthful, provide as many facts as are known, and communicate often to minimize fear. To avoid the "surprise" factor, whenever possible organizations can discuss the possibility of a merger or a demerger in more general terms to begin preparing people for the potential changes. People within the organization can keep themselves and others informed about the market forces that could lead to major changes such as a merger. It is important for members of any organization to be knowledgeable of the environment they work in and around, so they see that change may be needed to remain successful.

—Sherry Kwater

Whether Karen's intention was to squelch negative chatter about a major institutional change or to try to point out some type of positive outcome from a stressful transition ("be thankful you still have a job"), her comment only served to exacerbate the fears of her staff and to deter effective communication between leadership and front-line staff.

Had Karen responded to Ashley's wish for the merger to have "never happened" with a concerned request for further explanation, she would have shown her willingness to communicate with her staff and to understand their fears about how they would be affected by the merger—especially their personal anxieties about their own job security. A clear and complete understanding of their concerns would enable Karen to provide her staff with accurate information throughout the transition planning and implementation process. With this understanding, concerns about the reasons for the merger could be addressed with information about changing trends in the health care market and the effects on the local region that necessitated that changes be made at both institutions, resulting in the decision to merge. This could also be an opportunity to clearly share what the anticipated benefits to patients, communities, and the institutions and their employees might be. Rather than leaving the rumor mill unanswered, an open channel of communication could be used to acknowledge individuals' fears about the impact of this change on their own livelihoods (which may or may not be well-founded) and to provide for ongoing supportive dialogue to help staff members process what is expected to change and what will remain the same for them as individuals and as a work unit as the transition proceeds.

While effective communication can be the solution to many of the potential pitfalls encountered when trying to manage transitions and changes, evolving plans and decisions and the fears associated with change often make it difficult to identify and convey accurate and supportive information throughout an organization for the duration of the transition planning and implementation process. When decisions and information are continually evolving, as they always are in health care at all levels, there is often a precarious balance between waiting to communicate until information has been finalized in order to ensure accuracy and providing early information that is likely subject to change. It may even be tempting in a hectic environment to attempt to solve a seemingly straightforward problem by issuing a directive to change without any further communication at all.

–Donna Kandsberger

Reflection

Chances are, if you haven't gone through a merger or demerger so far, you will in the future. What day-to-day steps can be taken to proactively prepare your staff for such a possibility?

Even nurse managers feel anxious when confronted with a merger. How can you simultaneously support your staff *and* be sensitive to their anxieties while addressing your own?

Vignette 12.2: Easy Change

At St. Clara Hospital, nurse managers must obtain the approval of their nursing supervisor prior to discharging a patient. The policy was created when there was a problem managing empty beds and a physician complained to the CEO. Now, the director of nursing reasons, supervisors will know the status of a particular unit at all times.

"This is ridiculous," Dolores, one of the new nursing supervisors, tells a coworker. "All I basically do is acknowledge what the nurse managers tell me. The computer could easily do the same thing."

At the unit level, nurse managers are now requiring all nurses to "check in" with them prior to discharging a patient.

"It's stupid, I know," says Jill, a nurse manager. "It creates an extra step for everyone, but I guess we're all paying the price because a doctor blew his stack when his patient sat in the ED for 2 days, waiting to be admitted, when there was really an empty bed."

Expert Commentary: Vignette 12.2

Top-down change, like that discussed in this vignette, is rarely successful and usually adds unnecessary steps to existing processes. This type of change usually fails because the people who understand the process the best aren't involved in the solution. This type of forced change is typically met with a cynical response, especially when it creates more work and frustration for the individuals involved in doing the job. To create simple and effective workflows, the people performing the process in question must be involved. The more input people have in designing the change that affects their work, the more they will own the results. Leadership can describe the issues and boundaries of the decision-making and allow the people performing the work to suggest changes to resolve the complaint or issue. Leaders must provide people in the organization the knowledge and tools to create successful change activities.

Managing change is one of the most difficult and challenging areas for leadership teams. We live in a world that requires change to remain successful as a health care industry. Leadership can be proactive to prepare the organization for changes that are inevitable. A few of those changes include our attention to quality and safety, competition in the marketplace, the ability to rapidly embrace and implement evidence-based care, and positioning the organization for the financial realities facing hospitals and health systems today. Leaders must know their role during these periods of change:

- It is not the change that usually upsets people, it is the transition. It is the period of time when people are unsure how the change will affect them. They typically do not have the facts, and that creates anger and fear. The leader's role is to communicate as much detail as possible to the people affected by the change. Communicate often, and use multiple forms of communication such as verbal, memo, video, PowerPoint, newsletters, text messages, and individual conferences as examples. Communication is the most important tool for leadership.

- Ask for the guiding principles on how people will be treated during the change process. If roles will be eliminated, what process will be used to determine who stays in a role and who does not? Is it decided by seniority, knowledge or expertise, or performance evaluations, to name a few criteria?

- Listen carefully to what people are talking about. Never make them feel like their comments are silly. People work through the change process differently; there is not a right or wrong way. Never make promises or try to convince people the change is good. They will come to their own conclusions on whether the change is good or bad for them. Communicate the facts.

- Allow people time to process the information and vent their feelings and concerns. You cannot rush people to accept change before they are ready. Some change activities just take time. (It takes 9 months to have a baby, no matter how many people you put on the job!)

- Always reinforce what is known and communicate when and how the unknowns will be addressed. Even if all the answers are not known, it is important to keep people in the loop of the most current information. They need to be part of the process.

- It helps to have leaders highly visible during times of change, especially if they can be available during different times, shifts, and days of the week. People must feel they have direct access to leadership.

- Remain calm and positive. Leadership will set the tone for the change. If you are frustrated by the change, your staff will likewise be frustrated—and confused. As a leader, you must understand your own emotions related to the change. Your role is to be sure your staff has the facts, not the emotion.

- Provide education, knowledge, and tools to people. To be involved in a meaningful dialogue about a major change, they need to know how to provide input that will be viewed as useful in the change process.

The employees at St. Clara Hospital lack engagement. In organizations with a high degree of trust, you will also see a high degree of employee engagement throughout the organization. Their involvement is critical in the design of new processes, in the refinement of processes that have failed and led to complaints, and in assisting with understanding the cultural needs of the organization in times of major change. The people in the organization *are* the organization. As a leader, it is important to engage employees in the changes that will affect them. Employees will have a greater sense of ownership for the process when they are involved in the solution.

–Sherry Kwater

Top-down directives regarding policies and procedures can sometimes be effective, as in situations in which procedures must be performed in a specific and uniform manner or when subordinates are either unable or unwilling to take responsibility for particular decisions. However, as in this case, this type of directive can be counterproductive when front-line staff do not fully understand the reason for the directive—and even more so when they perceive the directive to be making the situation worse.

In this case, the director of nursing could have followed one of several courses of action. In all cases, the need for a solution to the problem surrounding tracking of bed status and its negative effect on patients awaiting admission must be clearly communicated to all levels of staff involved in bed tracking. In conjunction with this communication, the DON could, as in this scenario, decide on and implement a particular solution to the problem. Alternatively, she could enlist any combination of nursing supervisors, managers, and staff nurses to either recommend possible solutions for her to consider before making her decision or delegate authority to them to design and implement a solution. Involving the staff in the decision, whether as consultants or decision-makers, would increase their understanding and engagement in the issue and their sense of mutual ownership of the problem and commitment to working to achieve an effective solution.

One particularly powerful element informing the attitudes and behaviors of nurses is that of best interests of patients. Patients are the reason that nurses chose to be nurses. Promoting an understanding of how particular decisions or changes are oriented to provide the best possible care to patients is very often the best strategy to combat negativity and to motivate nurses to put aside differences, to temper their own needs in relation to those of the patients, and even to become involved in a positive manner in working toward solutions that will benefit patients.

–Donna Kandsberger

Reflection

How powerful are the nurse managers in your institution? For example, if all the managers joined together and went to higher administration with a plan for revising a policy like the one described earlier, what would happen?

What strategies can you use to balance the powers of medicine and nursing? That is, if a physician changes a patient-care policy, what role do nurses play in making the change happen (or not)?

If you have the ability to set policies for your own unit, what is your process? Do you get staff involved? How involved are your staff in day-to-day decision-making and problem-solving?

Summary

Rousseau and Tijoriwala (1999) describe factors that influence the willingness or hesitancy employees have toward change. First, and perhaps most important, is trust. Good managers work on building trust with their staff daily, not only when a crisis arises. Transparency, reliability, and advocacy are all part of the skill set effective nurse managers will use to develop trust between themselves and their staff. This, in turn, builds a foundation for smoother implementation of new policies and procedures.

These authors also describe how the perceived legitimacy of the new policy facilitates or inhibits implementation. If you, the nurse manager, consider a proposed or actual new policy as long overdue, you will create an environment on your unit that welcomes the change. If, however, you are opposed to the new process, it's likely your staff will convey the same attitude. The more that information can be shared about the rationale for policy change or implementation, the more likely nurses at all levels are to accept it. A "force-fed" change that is dictated by higher management is likely to meet resistance from both you and the rest of your staff.

Another consideration regarding change is the "psychological contract" that exists between employees and employers. Every individual in an institution has expectations and beliefs about what his or her work life entails. For example, employees expect that they will receive their paychecks promptly and reliably. When new policies are proposed that appear to violate the psychological contract, resistance and negativity will result. As a nurse manager, finding out what your staff expects from you and your institution can help make unspoken beliefs and expectations explicit, as well as decrease tension.

Activities

Establish a rotating advisory council to interface between you and the staff. The idea is twofold:

- To give staff an accessible resource to discuss, question, and constructively debate institutional policies and other concerns

- To give you, the nurse manager, an insider's perspective on what staff think and to help you build relationships

Be sure all staff members know that they can bring something to the advisory council anonymously, and that nobody will be "dinged" for speaking with the council.

Alternatively, establish a secure suggestion box for positive suggestions on how to improve the work climate on your unit. Provide guidelines on what constitutes "positive suggestions" and "work climate."

Or, make a list of the things that constitute your "psychological contract," whether reasonable or not. Go down the list and circle those items that are already part of your organization's operating policies. For the items not on your list, try to determine if they can be made into realistic goals or if they are blocking your ability to thrive professionally. You could do this same activity with your staff to get a feeling for the group mind-set.

13 | nurse managers as the problem

Recently, Hader (2010) reported on the results of a global assessment of nurse leaders that gave insight into some demographics about nurse managers. Obtaining survey input from nurse managers around the world, the analysis revealed that most were female, worked in hospitals or health systems, had more than 20 years of experience, and were the primary income for their family. Both Hispanics and African-Americans were underrepresented in the leadership domain. The 8.5% of respondents who were male were more likely to have moved into management at a young age. Regardless of which area of management they functioned in, men made more money than women for the same job. One of the leading complaints presented on the questionnaire was the need to juggle quality of care with financial metrics. Completing mandated paperwork was also a source of tension.

Nurse managers often find themselves unprepared for leadership. They may be staff one day and management the next, expected to supervise nurses with whom they once worked side by side. In our survey of blogs, many nonmanagerial nurses described conflicts that arose out of poor leadership. These conflicts included:

- **Not addressing cliques and alliances:** As a result, exclusion and other bad behaviors not only continue, but become the norm for anyone new entering the unit.

- **Not being a real presence on unit:** The nurse manager is never there when certain coworkers refuse to answer call bells or are playing Solitaire on the computer. This means staff can get away with poor practice or downright laziness.

- **Focusing on the negative:** Instead of saying, "Our nosocomial infection rate is one of the lowest in the institution," the manager will frame it as, "The numbers came out, and our unit had X number of ventilator-associated pneumonias last year."

- **Outright bullying of staff by the nurse manager:** This might be because the nurse manager is threatened by certain individuals, going through difficulties at home, under pressure from higher-ups, or a mean girl grown up. In their online survey of 303 nurses, Vessey, DeMarco, Gaffney, and Budin (2009) found that about 69% had experienced some form of bullying and aggression, with nurse managers and charge nurses accounting for a third of the aggression.

- **Using performance evaluations to retaliate against employees:** With the right ammunition, a nurse manager can make a bedside nurse look inefficient when, in reality, the nurse is taking the time to give good patient care.

- **Having favorites:** Just having favorites is distressing, but it's particularly distressing when nurse managers give favorite nurses their vacation requests and other favors at the expense of others.

At the same time, nurse managers are struggling with myriad conflicts that may transcend administrative levels. Regan and Rodriquez (2011) surveyed 42 nurse managers and assistant nurse managers working in a diverse hospital setting to uncover work values and supports. More than 80% of respondents had less than 3 years' experience as managers, and fewer than half felt empowered to carry out the work assigned to them. Support and resources for effective leadership of staff nurses were often missing as well.

Lee, Spiers, Yurtseven, Cummings, Sharlow, Bhatti, and Germann (2010) delivered a leadership program to 86 nurse managers and compared pre- and postintervention scores as well as conducting 18 face-to-face focus groups. They found that after completing the leadership program, nurse managers increased their ability to inspire others, but a negative impact on in work life and cynicism also occurred.

Okey Eneh, Vehvilainen-Julkunen, & Kvist (2012) polled 1,497 nurses to explore their thoughts on desirable qualities of nurse managers. Most of the group gave managers favorable marks for ethical and professional-development behaviors. When addressing relational abilities, nurse managers got good endorsements for using the staff's skills effectively. However, only half of the respondents felt they received constructive and helpful feedback from their manager.

Commentator Victoria Schirm addresses the problem of conflict from the nurse manager's perspective:

Clearly, nurse managers need the skill set for making sound decisions using respectful, nonjudgmental approaches. Rather than responding to incidents with preconceived impressions, nurse managers need to avoid conclusions and entrapment in others' emotions. In circumstances where viewpoints are varied, confronting bad behavior with even more dissension assumes that a villain exists or at the very least, there are victims who need to be rescued.

Threatening disciplinary action for policy transgressions or taking a stand on one side or another assume a conclusion that may not be accurate when all viewpoints are heard.

Too often, when concerns arise about a coworker, the issues are not shared directly with the persons involved. Consequently, the disagreements continue unabated. Nurse managers are in a position to make a positive difference when they take ownership and help others present their concerns in a transparent and respectful environment. As leaders, they can make a difference in promoting employee performance that, in turn, improves patient care and safety.

Smith (2011) encourages nurse managers to adopt the transformational leadership model, which is based on the need to constantly adapt and change as the health care domain changes. She describes leaders like this as good communicators, inspiring to others, trustworthy, and able to engage stakeholders. This kind of manager is adept at addressing conflict in the workplace by preventing much of it from ever occurring.

Vignettes, Commentaries, and Reflective Thinking

The remainder of this chapter presents vignettes about nurse managers being the problem, commentaries about the experiences represented in the vignettes, and opportunities to explore or reflect on the material.

Vignette 13.1: The "In" Crowd

Grace, an RN and certified diabetes educator, hangs out with other nurse specialists in the hospital, even though most of her day is spent with staff and patients on the medical unit. When Grace needs information or help, she turns to the medical nurses. When her job is done on their floor, however, she makes it clear she prefers to be with the group of clinical specialists who eat together in the cafeteria.

"It's like they're the popular girls in high school," Danielle, an RN on the medical unit, observes. "She and I were in the lunch line together, and she dumped me in a flash when she saw that they were already at a table."

Greta, the nurse manager on the medical unit, won't speak to Grace about her lack of courtesy and respect to the floor nurses because she and Grace go to the same church, and Greta considers Grace to be a friend of sorts. Greta also wants to stay in the good graces of the clinical specialists, because they have influence on important hospital committees.

Expert Commentary: Vignette 13.1

An important aspect of the educator role is establishing rapport with staff. Grace may not realize she is jeopardizing that relationship by ditching staff when the work on the floor is done. Grace needs honest feedback to understand how she is presenting herself and to build collegial relationships. Ideally, this is a dialogue between Grace and the staff—not necessarily with Greta's involvement. Greta could provide support for the staff member to discuss this with Grace directly.

If direct communication is not possible, then it will be up to Greta to engage Grace in problem-solving as a peer, especially if she is not Grace's supervisor. She can start by finding out how Grace feels she is doing in her role as educator. Questions to ask might include the following:

- How does Grace feel she is relating to staff?

- What obstacles is Grace encountering?

Greta needs to establish the ground rules for communication between them, drawing the distinction between their relationship at church and their roles at work. Greta's job is to prevent small issues from becoming big problems. Greta could state that she has noticed that Grace seems to prefer socializing with the CNS group, and that this is off putting for staff who would like to socialize with Grace as well. Greta can emphasize that she is interested in everyone's success and comfort on the unit, including Grace's. It will be important to listen carefully to Grace's response. Greta can then provide the support Grace needs to establish a more collegial relationship with staff.

–Kathleen Merrill Jackson

A large part of nursing professionalism is separating your personal life and issues from your professional practice. In this scenario, it seems as though Grace's personal friendships with the other nurse specialists are affecting her professional relationships with the nurses she works with on her unit. Additionally, the nurse manager, Greta, has allowed her personal relationship with Grace outside of work to prevent her from dealing with this situation directly. By separating their personal and professional lives, these issues may have been avoided entirely.

The development of cliques seems to occur naturally in work environments with a large population of women (e.g., nursing). In my experience, it can be extremely beneficial to have several male nurses on staff to help buffer the development of female cliques, which can be disruptive to professional relationships.

In summary, setting aside personal issues and incorporating more male nurses on staff can go a long way toward deterring cliques, which can be destructive to nursing relationships and morale.

–Deana Deeter

Reflection

Cliques are considered to be a high school behavior that involves women. How would you compare the "good old boy" network with female "cliques" in your organization?

What drives clique behavior? Do you believe that men are the solution to ending such behavior, or is there a deeper cause?

In your organization, do nurse managers have a clique? How do you work to prevent in-group and out-group behaviors among your peers?

Vignette 13.2: Missing Leadership

Teresa works the evening shift on the orthopedic floor. She is tired of coworkers and support staff spending their downtime surfing the Internet, checking their Facebook accounts, and making personal calls.

"It's ridiculous," she tells Eric, the nurse manager for the floor. "I'm answering call bells and taking care of their patients, while they have a great time goofing off in the station. Last night, a family member came and found me in a patient's room, because he couldn't get any of the nurses out at the station to answer a question for him."

Eric assures her he will "take care of it" and asks the evening supervisor to check the orthopedic floor periodically. Rachel, the evening supervisor, calls the floor twice to see how things are going on the evening shifts during the week after Eric talks to her and tells the unit secretary when she will be coming up to "make rounds."

The staff becomes adept at figuring Rachel out and manage to "make busy" during her visits. In between, however, they continue to let Teresa do the heavy lifting on the floor while they congregate in the station.

Expert Commentary: Vignette 13.2

Eric needs to stand by his word and "take care of it." It would be best if Eric conducted these surprise visits himself. Seeing his evening staff in action would enable him to make an accurate assessment of the issue. Aside from the basic unfairness to Teresa, there are HIPAA and basic privacy concerns when family members are driven to enter another patient's room to find a nurse. A team meeting with the evening staff to discuss issues and improve response to patient needs would be an important first step for Eric to take. The creation of a sense of team is important, so that work is a shared responsibility. The staff could plan to better meet patient needs and create a code of conduct that all sign. Eric needs to continually emphasize that all staff will be held accountable to this plan of action.

—Kathleen Merrill Jackson

The nurse manager in this scenario handled this situation very poorly. He sent an off-shift nursing supervisor, who may or may not have a direct affiliation to the unit, to do his "dirty work." Rachel's approach to the situation, making announced visits to the unit on an off shift, will do little to deter this behavior in the future.

It is critical for nursing leadership to have a regular presence on their unit(s) to hold staff accountable for their practice and to deter lazy behavior. It should not be a shock to nursing staff to see nursing leadership on their unit. If nurse managers are making only sporadic appearances on their unit(s), they are viewed as being out of touch with the issues of the unit and unavailable to staff. Regular presence by a nurse manager on the unit goes a long way toward gaining the trust and respect of staff members.

This situation would have more effectively been handled directly by the nurse manager himself. He would need to plan to make regular appearances on all shifts on the unit to stay attuned to the issues faced by nursing staff and to discourage negative behaviors on the unit.

–Deana Deeter

Reflection

What policies do you have in place regarding the use of the Internet during work time? Would you favor the installation of software that prohibited your staff from accessing the web?

How much time do you spend "policing" your staff to see if they use the Internet during their work time? Is it appropriate for nurse managers to do so?

What portion of your workday is spent sending and receiving emails? How do you handle emails that may have upsetting content?

Vignette 13.3: Shortcomings Rather Than Strengths

Missy receives a report on the incidence of nosocomial infections on her postsurgical floor. It notes that "In the last year, there were 10 infections that occurred which were identified as 'nosocomial.' We encourage you to be aware of this information and share it with nurses on your floor."

Throwing the paper down, she turns to Addison, one of the RNs who works with her. "Ten infections? What does that mean?"

Addison shrugs. "Who knows? We always get slapped on the knuckles by management. They could tell us: 'Hooray! You decreased infections by 10%.' Instead, they put everything so negatively."

"You're right. We never hear about the good things, or get good news. Just the bad stuff," Missy agrees.

Expert Commentary: Vignette 13.3

Ten nosocomial infections is information that lacks context and is therefore meaningless, as the nurses clearly identify. Missy should go back to management and ask for clarification. Ten infections among how many patients treated? Over how long a time period? What time of year? What types of infections? Under what conditions? Did the infections occur before or after new protocols were enacted? These are only a few of the questions that require an answer before the information is useful.

When the 10 infections are placed in context, this information can then be conveyed in a positive manner that empowers the nurses to act on it. Infection control is a complex issue that does not belong to nursing alone, and it is unfair to imply that infections among patients are solely due to lapses in nursing care. Infection control is an interdisciplinary team responsibility, so reducing the infection rate requires that it be addressed on multiple levels. The nurses need context and empowerment to address this issue in partnership with infection control, doctors, visitors, housekeepers, and everyone else who interacts with patients. It's important for nurses to have input into suggested solutions and how these will be enacted and enforced.

–Kathleen Merrill Jackson

As is the case with this vignette, hospital and nursing leadership often report quality metrics to staff on an annual or semiannual basis. This information is rarely provided in context (e.g., compared to other hospitals' infection rates or the hospital's historical rates). It is difficult to achieve nursing buy-in to affect quality metrics with sporadic reporting of data. Nurses are not inclined to change their practice if they are not aware there is a problem. Therefore, ongoing reporting of quality metrics with a target rate (or other unit of measure) is critical to keep staff informed of quality issues affected by their practice.

One strategy to generate enthusiasm and interest in quality improvement would be to identify a staff champion who is focused on a quality measure so that nursing staff receives feedback from a peer rather than data handed down by nursing leaders who are removed from bedside practice. Additionally, it is important to celebrate successes (e.g., a 10% decrease in infections) to generate momentum among staff members as they work toward the quality goal.

Active nursing participation in quality improvement activities is best achieved using a team approach, with direct involvement of staff nurses working collaboratively with nursing leadership. Ongoing reporting of QI data helps to keep practice issues that affect quality metrics in the forefront of nurses' minds and to demonstrate that changes in their clinical practice can make a difference in patient outcomes.

–Deana Deeter

Reflection

While one of your responsibilities is to ensure quality of patient care, what strategies do you use to present feedback to your staff members on their performance and patient outcomes?

Where do you draw the line between empowering your staff with needed information and motivating them to improve their performance in specific areas? How often do you give those who work for you a pep talk or word of encouragement?

What aspects of QI are your staff involved in? Are they expected to monitor their own performance and seek remediation if needed, or are you the person responsible?

Vignette 13.4: Bully Boss

As a staff nurse working in an outpatient clinic and looking forward to the arrival of a new unit manager, I soon found myself terribly disappointed. I had hoped for leadership with a commitment to patient care, but within 30 days, each clinic nurse and nurse practitioner was called into the manager's office. We were told we were lazy and worthless.

Our unit manager regularly yelled at us in front of physicians, other staff, and patients. When I defended a fellow nurse, I was told I was a liar. Although the medical director was present, this person said nothing. Some nurses were given the "silent treatment." This behavior frequently was directed to the senior, veteran nurse. The unit manager informed us that she was informed by senior management that the future priority of the clinic was to seek "younger and cheaper help." Nurses who witnessed these events were not prepared to support their senior colleagues for fear that they would be the next victim.

The unit manager's tirade continued in staff meetings. Questions were received with demeaning and belittling responses. She would roll her eyes at new ideas. Additionally, she sent nasty and demeaning emails and even challenged the credentials of nurse practitioners. She encouraged others to turn against each other and attempted to destroy established interdepartmental relationships.

These experiences were devastating to the morale and the cohesiveness of the clinic. Staff reacted by working and caring less. Some nurses began to lash out at other nurses. Many of us felt that we could not function at our best level when we had become increasingly nervous or agitated. The fact was that the unit manager was a bully.

Some of us attempted to report the new unit manager's incivility, but we were blocked by the director of nursing from pursuing these issues through the normal channels. The director of nursing had witnessed the behaviors. Whatever measures were there for dealing with this issue were clearly inadequate. There was a covert acceptance of bullying. I am afraid health care organizations tolerate incivility because it has a low probability of consequences for their bottom line.

I left after 9 months. It was the bullying and constant negativity that drove me out of the facility. I was sad about this but felt helpless to change it.

–Anonymous

Expert Commentary: Vignette 13.4

If the director of nursing fails to respond, then the chief executive officer of the hospital would be the last resort. Under these conditions, a nurse has only three options:

- Try to change the situation through the chain of command.

- Stay and try to change the culture from within.

- Quit and answer exit interview questions honestly.

To address the issue in the chain of command, it is important that the nurse files a complaint rather than verbally complain. In other words, document incidences of abuse and bullying behavior. The documentation should be as objective, complete, and unemotional as the documentation of patient behavior would be. It's appropriate to remind leadership that the manager's behavior violates Joint Commission standards. Detailed documentation, including date, time, and witnesses present, should provoke a response from the director of nursing or CEO. If not, the nurse may have no choice but to leave.

A wise nursing leader creates a team by setting clear guidelines for communication, treating staff as colleagues worthy of respect, and involving them in seeking solutions to problems. Mutual goal setting and codes of conduct to which all staff and managers commit can be helpful if all are held accountable. In complex environments, leadership is emergent and dynamic among team members.

Successful teamwork requires that nursing leaders engage their followers to help shape the leadership of the unit together. To do this, nursing leaders must create a culture of psychological safety, where nurses can speak out and be heard without fear of retribution. In a psychologically safe culture, bullying cannot take root. This culture is one of mutual respect and holding each other accountable. With the assurance of psychological safety, nurses can have critical conversations with colleagues and managers with a shared goal of improving patient care and creating peace in the work environment.

–Kathleen Merrill Jackson

I think this vignette illustrates the importance of having strong, enforceable, institutional policies against bullying behaviors that are applicable to all staff, across all settings. In this situation, where attempts to report the unit manager's behavior were blocked by the director of nursing, I feel that staff is entitled to pursue further action outside of the normal department of nursing channels. This manager's behaviors were witnessed by physicians and the medical director, so reporting her behaviors through medical channels, or even through human resources, may prove more fruitful. It may also be worth collecting staff or even patients' examples of mistreatment or witnessed behavior prior to taking action outside of the department of nursing to support the case.

In summary, institutional policies against bullying should be in place and enforceable, without being punitive if staff escalate concerns to a higher level—even outside their immediate department.

–Deana Deeter

Reflection

Given the Joint Commission requirements on workplace behaviors and civility, what measures have you and your organization taken to make sure relationships on your unit are respectful and courteous?

Reflect on your last week at work and your interactions with your staff. Having read this chapter, can you determine if your behavior could be labeled as bullying or relationally aggressive?

Does your body language (appearance, actions like sighing, rolling your eyes, frowning, and other nonverbal signs of your feelings) convey negative feelings toward your employees?

Vignette 13.5: Walking the Line/ Not Rocking the Boat

Janelle and Paul work in a large academic medical center. When there is a certain nurse vacancy rate, nurses who agree to work those shifts get paid extra. These shifts are called "bonus shifts."

Paul and his wife are about to buy a house, so Paul picks up a lot of bonus shifts to get the extra money. But recently, the extra pay that Paul should be getting for picking up bonus shifts has not been showing up in his paycheck. When Janelle asks him about it, Paul says, "I can't bring it up with management because I'm applying to graduate school, and I need a recommendation. It sucks, but I don't want to rock the boat."

Janelle is outraged on Paul's behalf and feels that the hospital is essentially stealing from Paul. Janelle says, "It's insane that a performance evaluation or a school recommendation can be used as a weapon against you like that!"

Expert Commentary: Vignette 13.5

Paul needs to speak with his manager about this immediately. It is both possible and probable that his not being paid is a benign oversight. He can ask his manager for assistance fixing the problem as opposed to accusing the manager of deliberately withholding pay. He should double-check his numbers to make sure that the pay is indeed missing, and then report that the money is not showing up in his paycheck, which is a simple fact. Finally, he can request a resolution. Bonus pay is a separate issue from the recommendation for graduate school. In addition, Paul needs to identify a management ally who will provide the recommendation now. He will get a better recommendation when he stands up for himself.

–Kathleen Merrill Jackson

This scenario suggests that a significant power differential exists between nursing leadership and nursing staff, in which management is seen as unapproachable, no matter what the situation. This creates an environment in which staff do not report problems, no matter how big or small, for fear of the personal repercussions. This can negatively affect patient safety and staff satisfaction on the unit.

Nursing leadership must be approachable to cultivate a culture of trust on the unit. Performance evaluations and recommendation letters highlight the positive accomplishments and qualities of staff and to raise the bar for future performance, rather than being used as a form of punishment.

Once again, regular presence of nursing leadership on the unit(s) helps to demonstrate to staff that leaders are available to them. This opens the lines of communication so that leaders are more aware of the issues on their unit(s).

–Deana Deeter

Reflection

How do you make yourself both available and "present" to really listen to issues your staff may experience? Are they more likely to come to you with concerns, or, after the fact, do you find out from someone else that an issue has occurred?

How supportive of each other are the nurse managers in your institution? Can you collaborate as a group to share solutions to common problems, or do you tend to avoid discussing any issues that may be bothering you?

Vignette 13.6: Sanctimonious Scheduling

The psych unit nurse manager, Lee Ann, has tried many different ways of scheduling vacations for the nurses on her floor, but someone always complains. This year, she posts a vacation sign-up sheet and asks the RNs to share their requests.

After spending hours trying to be fair in allocating first and second requests for vacations, Lee Ann posts the schedule. Nelly, one of the newer nurses, confronts Lee Ann in her office after seeing the schedule. "You've given all your favorites on day shift their first choices. I was told you looked out for your friends and gave them preferential treatment," Nelly says. Lee Ann can only look at her in shock and bewilderment, unable to explain that she rationed vacations according to choice and seniority.

Expert Commentary: Vignette 13.6

A review of the schedule will help Lee Ann determine if Nelly's accusations have any basis in fact. If so, Lee Ann should be aware of her unconscious bias in scheduling and can work to overcome it.

One solution might be to delegate scheduling to Nelly so she can experience the intricacies firsthand or teach the staff to do self-scheduling. Either way, Nelly could be put in charge of creating the schedule with final approval by Lee Ann. This is a teachable moment for Nelly and can create greater respect and honest communication between Lee Ann and Nelly. Lee Ann also needs to communicate that Nelly's lack of respect is unacceptable. Respectful feedback from Nelly can be requested along with strategies to offer it.

–Kathleen Merrill Jackson

The nurse manager in this scenario may benefit from being transparent about her strategy for scheduling vacations prior to soliciting to vacation requests to avoid being accused of playing favorites. It may also be useful to offer a formal process for nurses to challenge their schedule if they believe it to be unfair. Additionally, the nurse manager may be able to avoid blame for scheduling vacations if he or she delegates scheduling responsibilities to a scheduling committee of staff members who would approve a final schedule following self-scheduling by nursing staff.

In summary, processes such as staff self-scheduling may be beneficial in limiting the feeling of favoritism in scheduling among staff. Proactively sharing scheduling strategies (e.g., requests granted based on seniority, etc.) and including an avenue to challenge scheduling practices that seem unfair may also be helpful in empowering staff during the scheduling process.

–Deana Deeter

Reflection

Is it appropriate for nurse managers to have friendships with their staff? Why or why not? If you were a staff member on the unit you now manage, how was your relationship changed by moving into a management position?

Have you ever been accused of favoritism by your employees? What was or would be your response to such an accusation?

Summary

Nurse managers must have a diverse skill set, acting as both business person and caring coworker. Often, the preparation nurses receive for such leadership roles mostly consist of on-the-job training, which can result in feeling overwhelmed and unprepared. In such circumstances, bullying behaviors or relational aggression can occur, further increasing the tension. Becoming self-aware of your strengths and weaknesses as a leader can help you locate resources to continually improve your abilities without waiting to be told you need to make a change.

Relationships among coworkers are often unique to the nurse manager. Some managers feel comfortable socializing with their staff, while others maintain strict boundaries. Being viewed as unapproachable might lead your staff to avoid interacting with you any more than necessary, but being too friendly with your staff can create other kinds of problems.

Ultimately, the best teacher for a nurse manager is experience. Surrounding yourself with others who can mentor and support you is essential. Figuring out ways to de-stress will help you cope with inevitable on-the-job challenges. Whether you exercise, journal, sing, or read books as a way of relaxing and refreshing, take care of yourself first so you can be able to take care of others.

Activity

For 1 workweek, keep a journal on the conflicts, both big and little, that occur during your day. Keep it simple, but identify who, what, where, and when for each conflict (to the degree you can) and the emotion(s) you experienced at the time.

Allow another week to go by before you look back at your conflict journal. Then, sit down and see if you can figure out why each incident occurred. See if there are themes or patterns that are causing conflict, and note whether your management style and response are consistent across situations and people.

part V friction fallout

14 | patients as victims

Some units have a reputation for being toxic. These are the units that, when you arrive there, something just feels *off*—employees seem cynical about leadership, nurses don't treat each other well, and there's a general sense of frustration and hopelessness about the possibility for improvement. These units are usually terrible places to work. It's difficult—if not impossible—to have a happy, productive day at work when the environment in your workplace is so negative. So, clearly, a toxic culture negatively affects employees.

But one feature of a toxic environment that we may not think about as often or as readily is the negative impact on patients. When employees are unhappy at work, it can lead to a wide variety of negative patient consequences, as shown in the vignettes in this chapter. The Institute of Medicine (IOM) acknowledged this link in its 2005 report, *Keeping Patients Safe: Transforming the Work Environment of Nurses.* The IOM report indicates the threats to patient safety typical of the nursing work environment and that these threats are *caused* by organizational management practices, work design issues, and organizational culture (Institute of Medicine, 2005).

Heather Spence Laschinger and Michael Leiter (2006) recently conducted a study testing the hypothesis that nursing environments are linked with burnout and engagement, and that burnout and engagement were in turn linked with patient safety outcomes. They note that "the results are consistent with the notion that patient safety outcomes are associated with the quality of nursing practice work environment and the burnout/engagement process plays an important mediating role" (p. 265). They go on to say that the results indicate that when "nurses perceive that their work environment supports professional practice, they are more likely to be engaged in their work, thereby ensuring safe patient care" (Spence Laschinger & Leiter, 2006, p. 265). In sum, then, when the culture of a unit or organization is unhealthy, it negatively affects both patients and nurses.

There's an interesting ethics issue entwined in these findings that scholars don't usually talk about. When the medical teams' dysfunction negatively affects patient care, that means patients are more likely to fall, get bedsores, get nosocomial infections, or experience other adverse events. If *you* were a patient, wouldn't you prefer to be cared for in a unit where nurses supported each other, folks got along, and the culture was generally healthy?

Of course, we don't give patients this opportunity. Patients usually wind up wherever the ambulance drops them off or at whatever institution is geographically closest. We don't tell them, "Hey, watch out for the surgical ICU at General Public Institution! Those folks have a seriously messed-up culture down there!" And woe to the patient who winds up in the unit with a toxic work environment—as you've just seen, that patient is statistically significantly more likely to experience an adverse safety event. When you strip the politically correct language away, what we're really saying is this: Unhealthy hospital culture can kill patients.

So far, we've only talked about nurses *unintentionally* harming patients. But unfortunately, there are nurses out there who are more intentional about it. It's shocking to read blogs about nurses withholding pain medications, being rough with patients, and generally treating patients cruelly. For example, if a patient complains about a particular nurse, in the future, that nurse might be rough with that patient. Or consider a nurse who physically restrains a patient because the patient is a nuisance or annoying.

Recently, a clinical case occurred in our institution with a young patient in our neuroscience ICU. This young woman, despite being in a drug-induced coma, was incredibly active in bed. She was constantly moving, rolling over, and generally creating work for the nurses. Additionally, the patient had been in the hospital for almost 6 months—an incredibly long time. The nurses on the unit were burned-out to the max. In general, the culture in the neuroscience ICU was pretty good, but it was really being tested in this instance. In particular, the nurses had started to place four-point restraints on the patient. The nurse manager was concerned, because the patient didn't meet the hospital criteria for a patient who should be in restraints.

The moral of this story is that when nurses get fatigued and burned out, patient care suffers. Sometimes it suffers because a nurse is intentionally, maliciously trying to harm the patient (hopefully this is the exception to the rule), and sometimes it suffers because the nurse is unintentionally changing his or her behaviors as a coping mechanism.

So what can a nurse manager do to ensure that patients aren't victims? One strategy is to rotate difficult patients among nurses. When nurses get burned out taking care of a particular patient (such as the neuroscience ICU patient), the best course of action may be to get some new people involved. Explore whether the patient can be temporarily transferred to a different unit (perhaps the medical ICU) so that the nurses there can take care of him or her for a while.

On a more global level, it's critical for nurse managers to understand that culture affects patient outcomes. After that awareness has been developed, the nurse manager can try to take steps to improve the toxic culture in his or her unit, perhaps by increasing communication and respect or increasing role-modeling behaviors.

Vignettes, Commentaries, and Reflective Thinking

The remainder of this chapter presents vignettes about patients as victims, commentaries about the experiences represented in the vignettes, and opportunities to explore or reflect on the material.

Vignette 14.1: Painful Practice

Annie, a nurse on the evening shift of the surgical floor, is unhappy with her job and has a difficult personal life. Although she has gotten negative feedback in her evaluations about her interactions with patients, Annie doesn't change her ways. In particular, Annie withholds pain medication from postop patients, believing they might "get addicted to narcotics" (or so she says). Eventually, Tia, another evening nurse, goes to the nurse manager.

"Patients have been complaining about Annie. She won't give them postop pain meds on time, and she almost taunts them about even asking for it. It makes it hard for me to work with her. She's mistreating patients and giving our floor a bad reputation!"

The nurse manager, Katrina, tells Tia she will take care of the problem. She calls Annie in and tells her what Tia said, using Tia's name. Annie becomes irate and says Tia has a grudge against her. "She's just setting me up!" Annie insists.

That evening, at work, Annie confronts Tia in the locker room as their shift begins. "Thanks for being a tattletale! Now I'm in trouble with Katrina, and maybe I'll even lose my job. I hope you're satisfied." That evening, Annie is even rougher with her patients and retaliates against Tia at every opportunity.

Expert Commentary: Vignette 14.1

This vignette illustrates the importance of professionalism. Professionalism has become a business-school buzzword, but its real meaning, and thoughtful implementation, matters tremendously in nursing practice and health care in general.

Withholding pain medication from post-operative patients and taunting them when they ask for it are mean and petty behaviors—but they are also unprofessional. Part of a nurse's job is to deliver pain medication as ordered when patients ask for it. If a nurse refuses to do that, she's not doing her job. If she has serious concerns about addiction issues, then she needs to raise those concerns with the physicians ordering the meds, an

MD from palliative care, a pain specialist, or her nurse manager. Refusing to give patients narcotics is not an appropriate way to address concerns about opioid addiction.

The nurse manager's job in this situation is to ask Annie if she is in fact withholding narcotics from patients and then tell her that if so, she's not fulfilling the requirements of her job related to dispensing medications and appropriately relieving pain. The manager should then ask Annie why she withholds pain meds. If she's truly worried about addiction, then she could do an in-service with an NP or MD from palliative care to really learn about opioid addiction. If she's taking her work frustrations out on her patients, as Tia suspects, then the manager needs to have an empathic conversation with Annie about her work difficulties and see what possible solutions there are. She also needs to schedule regular follow-ups with Annie.

Telling Annie that Tia complained about her is likely to create a toxic work environment for both Tia and Annie, but is also unprofessional. Sorting out the truth of Annie's behavior is what matters. Turning it into an issue of who tattled on whom ignores the fact that Annie may not be giving her patients the care they need. The manager's focus needs to be on work, not personalities.

What's really missing here is leadership. Nurse managers need to remember that they are not just bureaucrats and enforcers of rules, they are also role models, example setters, and important supporters of staff nurses. A good manager does not have favorites, would never tell one nurse the name of a nurse who complained about her, and would make it clear that professional standards must prevail on the floor at all times. A good manager understands that nursing is a hard job, that working with other people inevitably leads to friction, and that part of managing is helping people see their way through their work conflicts and learn something from them, rather than just feeling criticized about whatever mistakes of protocol or policy they may have made.

Above all, nurse managers need to treat staff with respect and empathy while maintaining high standards of professionalism.

If nurses see that such behavior is expected and rewarded, they will find it easier to treat patients in the same way.

–Theresa Brown

There are multiple dynamics going on in this example. Annie is obviously struggling in many aspects of her life, and her professional performance is unsatisfactory on multiple levels. Annie is exhibiting unprofessional, unethical, and even aggressive behavior toward her patients and colleagues.

Withholding pain medications from postop patients is just one example. There are many complex barriers to effective pain management, some of which originate from the provider. This could be a case of simple mistaken knowledge, but given the other information provided about Annie, it is more likely that it is coupled with deeply held biases. These biases likely cloud Annie's ability to assimilate the factual information about the following:

- Postoperative pain

- The improved outcomes and decreased complications associated with the appropriate treatment of pain post-operatively

- The nature of addiction

- The evidence that postoperative pain treatment does not lead to addiction

These beliefs are also implicated in Annie's decisions to violate her professional and ethical obligation to treat patients' pain.

Annie's words and behavior also indicate that she has (or has developed) deeply ingrained cognitive mechanisms that enable her to disengage from personal responsibility for her behavior and instead assign blame to others (such as Tia and her patients). Her externalization of blame and lack of behavioral changes persist, despite negative evaluations. This pattern of coping is especially troubling, as it will likely mean a difficult remediation process that may be outside the scope of what is reasonable for her employer to fully support.

Tia is absolutely correct. Annie's behavior implicates the entire nursing staff and the floor's reputation. It appears that Katrina, the nurse manager, has not met her obligations to the nursing staff and to the patients in this case. The negative evaluations without subsequent negative consequences to Annie for repeated behavior have reinforced to Annie that she can continue in this pattern without any serious threat to her job. This also reinforces that her behavior is not terribly serious.

Katrina has also failed by giving Annie Tia's name during her discussion with Annie. This disclosure further enables Annie to assign blame, segment the issue to a problem with one other nurse, and amplify her already maladaptive behavior. Instead, Katrina could have met with Annie to discuss "complaints" she received about Annie's care in general and her failure to appropriately treat patients in pain. The failure to medicate patients could easily be determined by reviewing patient records and by following up with the patients themselves, when possible. Also, Katrina could have explored Annie's beliefs about pain control and addiction in a conversational manner. Given Annie's degree of disengagement, she may have voluntarily shared her beliefs about addiction in the postop period. This would have provided Katrina with a firsthand account with which to challenge Annie's behavior.

Nurses (and nurse managers) can sometimes be empathetic to a fault. Here, Katrina can understand some of the situational factors impairing Annie's ability to provide acceptable care without excusing the behavior. It is appropriate to refer Annie to outside care and counseling, but this must be done in conjunction with, rather than instead of, corrective action. It is also critical that Katrina be mindful of whether she is allowing herself to be bullied by Annie. Katrina herself may benefit from seeking assistance and guidance from a mentor in dealing with the difficulties of managing.

Katrina's primary obligation is to the well-being of the patients and the function of the nursing unit as a whole. Failure to take action when nursing care is subpar and unethical is dangerous to patients. It is also seriously detrimental to the organizational health of the nursing unit because it demoralizes the other nurses, sends a message that care need not be acceptable, and discourages open communication between the nurses and Katrina. This is especially true given Annie's pattern of aggression and bullying to quiet her coworkers. Katrina must defeat the effectiveness of Annie's bullying.

Katrina must establish a clear and factual framework for Annie's behavior going forward. Next, she can initiate corrective action that is appropriate to the totality of Annie's behavior over time and establish expectations for behavior and consequences for a deviation from the behavior in a completely transparent manner. It may be appropriate for Katrina to directly supervise Annie's work for a time. It is certainly appropriate for Katrina to regularly audit Annie's care and to act consistently with the previously established consequences.

Annie will either slowly work to correct her behavior, or her continued behavior will result in serious consequences, including termination if warranted. No manager takes pleasure in placing someone on corrective action. Strong and consistent adherence to standards that value appropriate nursing care will improve not only individual nursing performance but positively affect the morale and function of the nursing unit.

–Kelly Dineen

Reflection

What is your personal philosophy about administration of pain medication for patients? Are there situations where you feel it's appropriate to withhold pain medication or give the least amount possible? Do you err on the side of believing patient reports of pain or on the side of being cautious about drug-seeking, addictive behavior?

What feedback do you give to nurses who do not treat patients in pain with prompt medications? Patients report that their pain is chronically underrated. How can you make sure that your patients do not feel they receive subpar pain treatment?

Vignette 14.2: Family Friction

Aria, an RN with 10 years of experience on a medical-surgical floor at Community Hospital, has worked a double shift after another nurse calls off sick. After 10 hours of caring for difficult patients, she is tired and grouchy.

A patient, Mr. Truman, is recovering from major abdominal surgery. He needs a dressing change and pain medication, but Aria is busy helping another patient who has IVs and mobility problems get to the bathroom. Mrs. Truman searches her out. "My husband really needs you," she tells Aria. "He's got a lot of pain."

"I'll be there as soon as I can," Aria replies.

Ten minutes later, Mrs. Truman shows up again, repeating her request. This time, Aria follows her down the hall and tells Mr. Truman she is getting his meds and the supplies for his dressing change. Aria completes her care of Mr. Truman but is rough and unpleasant as she does so, because she feels stressed and unappreciated. Mrs. Truman later files a complaint with Aria's nurse manager.

Expert Commentary: Vignette 14.2

The impossibility of one nurse needing to be in two places at once comes up over and over again in clinical practice, and it's actually an easily solved problem. Answering call lights should be everyone's responsibility, and there should be enough staff on the floor that Aria could call an aide, another nurse, or even the nurse manager to either help the patient get to the bathroom or give the pain medication to Mr. Truman. Managers also need to be tuned in to whether nurses are working a double shift and be prepared to give an overtired nurse more backup.

The real problem here is the chronic one of hospitals not having enough staff to cover call-offs and expecting nurses on the floor to make up the difference without any negative consequences to themselves or patients. Aria is only human; being confronted in the hallway by an irate family member is likely to produce irritation and a feeling of being unappreciated, even if the complaints are legitimate.

The nurse manager will need to hear out Mrs. Truman's complaint and then apologize for not staffing the floor adequately and not giving Aria the support she needed to do her job. She also needs to follow up with Aria in a supportive way, making clear that being rough with patients is, of course, not OK but admitting that Aria was overworked.

–Theresa Brown

Aria's behavior is all too common in nursing. At least one primary factor here is that Aria is not mindful of her own capacity, needs, and limits. This is the classic tale of the "burned-out" nurse. The same traits and strengths that may lead individuals into nursing in the first place can easily become distorted and negatively affect performance. Nurses often have a strong desire to help others as well as advanced abilities to empathize and sacrifice for the greater good. Many nurses can balance these traits with self-care and reflection. However, achieving that balance takes meticulous attention that is often difficult. Nurses often volunteer for extra shifts despite their need for rest, because their desire to help is stronger. These selfless qualities are often exploited by institutions trying to solve staffing difficulties and colleagues with other motives, ranging from getting a day off to seeking companionship for their own out-of-balance state. Nurses have to take time to recharge and reflect, or they will have little in the way of valuable care to offer others.

Aria may be distorting reality, or she may in fact not be appreciated by her institution or even by the Trumans. That reality does not justify taking out the associated frustrations on a patient. Good nursing performance requires the ability to provide consistent and appropriate care, even in the absence of appreciation. This is why it is so critical for nurses to be self-evaluative and to develop strategies for identifying their feelings and separating those from their behavior.

This vignette does not indicate whether Aria has a pattern of this behavior. It is possible that this incident was out of character and represents a breaking point for her. It is a warning sign for Aria, and it may be an opportunity for change.

Patients (and their families) are in vulnerable positions by virtue of their illness (or concern for a loved one). Understandably, they may be short on patience or have an altered sense of time. It is not surprising that Mrs. Truman sought out Aria more than once. Caregivers are evaluating patient needs in the context of their universe of patient experiences. Individual patients are evaluating their needs in the context of their own experience.

There were several missed opportunities to prevent a negative response from the Trumans. Aria could have validated Mrs. Truman's concerns during the first request, rather than responding the way she did. Aria could also have asked another nurse to give Mr. Truman his pain medication or another employee on the floor to help the other patient with mobility issues.

Sometimes there is just no additional help, and it doesn't sound like Aria was in a position to drop what she was doing with the patient with mobility issues. Aria still had an opportunity to ameliorate the situation, however, by apologizing to Mr. Truman for the delay, treating him respectfully, and validating his frustration and pain. Aria could have given Mr. Truman the pain medication and then returned later to change his dressing once the medication had taken effect. The level of pain probably enhanced the perception that Aria was rough with him. Thereafter, if Aria planned ahead for his next dose of pain medication, as well as checking on him more frequently than absolutely necessary to assess his pain, it would reassure both of the Trumans that help was nearby.

As a side note, when talking to patients and their families, it is never acceptable to take out frustrations on them, nor is it their responsibility to accommodate or understand issues with staffing or high acuity. These issues should never be offered up to patients as a reason or excuse for delay. Patients want to be cared for, and they may want and should be offered an apology if they feel they are not receiving adequate attention. They can't be expected to understand the demands on or empathize with the nurse. Sharing that information may make patients angry. Worse, it could have a chilling effect on patient complaints out of fear of "bothering" the nurses. That attitude could lead to delay in detecting complications because patients do not report new or increased symptoms. This could also lead to other consequences such as falls, because patients may try to manage their own needs rather than call for help.

Aria's manager has an obligation to meet with Aria and explore the situation. If this is the first incident of this kind, the manager could encourage Aria to take a few days off to recharge and also encourage employee assistance or other counseling to assist Aria in developing coping strategies for dealing with the stressors that have lead her to act out toward a patient.

–Kelly Dineen

Reflection

If you are not physically present when issues occur between patients and their families and your staff, how can you respond to troublesome situations?

What information about your unit are patients and their family members given on admission? Have you ever sensed that there are unreal expectations between visitors and your staff?

How could your staff respond in situations like the one above? Can you count on them to cover for each other, or would they end up in similar circumstances?

Vignette 14.3: Power Trip

Lily works with Wayne, an RN who is the only male nurse in the entire OR. He has been there since Lily started 5 years ago, and Lily gets the sense that Wayne is on a major power trip. Lily says to Nancy, another nurse on the unit, "Every morning, Wayne bosses all of the RNs around, even though he's not our manager and was, in fact, passed over for the position. Most of us just ignore him, but when he starts treating patients roughly, I get upset."

Nancy replies, "I know what you mean! Wayne loves to get the extra warm blanket for patients, but then he'll stand there with the blanket and talk to someone else while the patient is shivering. I've seen him do this so many times it has to be deliberate."

Lily knows that no patient has ever complained about Wayne, which she finds really surprising. Despite this, Lily and Nancy are disgusted with his behavior. They don't know what to do, because their manager likes Wayne and frequently turns to him for advice.

Expert Commentary: Vignette 14.3

It's hard to tell in this situation if the problem is Wayne being on a power trip or Lily and Nancy not liking him. The other problem is that Lily and Nancy aren't sure whether their manager will hear their complaints against Wayne or if he's considered a favorite and can't be criticized.

Let's say Lily and Nancy *do* go to the manager and describe Wayne's waiting to give patients blankets. The manager needs to hear them out and promise to keep an eye on the situation but affirm that no patients have ever complained about Wayne. This suggests that Lily's and Nancy's perception of the problem may be more severe than the patients'.

The manager will also need to probe further and attempt to discover what's at the root of Lily's and Nancy's complaint. If Wayne does boss the other nurses around, then that's a cause of concern, because it will make them resent him.

The difficulty here is sorting out the legitimate complaints from what we might call "artifacts of resentment." Wayne's acting like a leader when he isn't is not appropriate at work, so are the blankets really the issue? The manager's challenge is to stay open-minded and empathic, while also being fair to Wayne, Lily, and Nancy.

—Theresa Brown

This vignette represents a type of situation that may be very difficult for nurses to manage. It is hard for any person to deal with an individual like Wayne in the workplace. It may be even more difficult for nurses, because nurses tend to be natural helpers and want to be liked. Therefore, they are less likely to confront their coworkers. In addition, the workplace depends heavily on collaboration; there is a natural fear that confrontation will break down that collaboration. Wayne's behavior probably requires pushback from both his colleagues and his manager.

Nonetheless, Lily and Nancy are letting Wayne's behavior affect their workplace. There are actually three behaviors they have identified as problematic:

- Wayne bosses all the RNs around, even though he is not in charge.

- Wayne is rough with patients.

- Wayne insists on getting warm blankets but does not give them to the patients promptly.

Of these, the third is the easiest to remedy. Lily and Nancy should simply anticipate the need for warm blankets and bring them to the patient on their initial assessment. It isn't clear whether Wayne is simply easily distracted or engaging in purposeful behavior, and Nancy's conclusion that it is deliberate may be accurate or it may be a cognitive distortion of mindreading in which we all engage from time to time. If Lily or Nancy observes the behavior again, they have an opportunity to model appropriate assertive behavior for their colleagues by simply reminding Wayne publicly that the patient is still waiting for the blanket.

They also have an opportunity to model appropriate behavior in dealing with the first issue. Ignoring Wayne does not seem to be sending the message to him that his colleagues do not appreciate his actions. Depending on the issue, they may be able to use a passive approach to send the message gently without embarrassing him. (Note: This author is not advocating passive behavior in a maladaptive way, but suggesting that it can be used strategically in some situations.) They could ask him if he is the charge nurse today in a clarifying way. They could also take one of his ideas to the charge nurse or manager by saying something like, "Wayne, that is an interesting approach. Let's see if the charge nurse thinks that will work."

The second issue, roughness with patients, is the most concerning. Again, if the nurses observe the behavior, they could approach the bedside and say something like, "Wayne, I think you ate your Wheaties today. You rolled this gentleman over more forcefully than I think you realized," and then ask the patient if he is OK. That would diffuse some of Wayne's power over the patient, open up an opportunity for the patient to acknowledge the rough behavior, and call Wayne on the behavior at the same time.

If the passive confrontation approaches don't seem to work, Wayne may need to be assertively confronted. For example, if Wayne is bossing several nurses around in the morning, Lily or Nancy could say, "Wayne, I appreciate that you have a lot of experience here and want to help, but the way you are talking to me is offensive. It makes me feel like you don't trust me to care for the patient. I would not treat you that way, and I am asking you not to treat me that way."

This is not easy, and takes a great deal of moral courage. Therefore, the nurses will need the support and encouragement of their manager. Lily and Nancy can't assume that the manager won't act because they perceive that the manager likes Wayne. The manager should listen and decide on a best course of action, no matter how much he or she may like Wayne. Also, the manager may consult Wayne strategically. Despite Wayne's behavior, he may have good ideas that the manager appreciates. The nurse manager may also do it to give him a measure of control that is obviously important to him. Consulting him likely reduces his need to act out to grasp at power. On the other hand, he or she may not have observed Wayne's bullying behavior directly. In either case, it is important to approach the manager with the issue in a factual manner and with a strategy in hand. The manager can continue monitoring the situation to ensure that Lily and Nancy are not engaged in their own maladaptive, bullying response to Wayne.

–Kelly Dineen

Reflection

What word would you use to describe the relationships among your staff? To what degree do you feel the quality of their interactions is reflective of your management style?

If you observe a staff member being rude or aggressive to a patient or coworker, how do you respond? Do you feel confident in your ability to handle this type of conflict?

As a nurse manager, how might you help guide nurses who want to be part of the leadership on your unit?

Vignette 14.4: Nurses as Victims

Sabrina is a nurse in a busy urban emergency department. One night after work, as she is talking with her husband and telling him about her day, she says, "You know, it's really incredible the way patients treat me. I mean, I realize they often have to wait an insanely long time before they actually get seen and that the waiting room is crowded, smelly, and genuinely unpleasant, but some days I feel like a literal punching bag for patient dissatisfaction."

Sabrina continues telling her story. "Tonight, I was taking care of a man who came to the ED because he was experiencing chest pain. Turns out, it was just acid reflux, and we were arranging to discharge him when the guy took me by the shoulders and shook me, hard, in his effort to convince me that it wasn't just acid reflux."

Sabrina's husband is upset that patients are physically harming Sabrina at work, and he wonders what management is going to do about it. Sabrina replies, "Well that's the real kicker! When I told my nurse manager about it, she was totally unsupportive.

She told me that patient abuse is just part of the role in the ED, and I should just get used to it. I mean, how is that helpful?"

Expert Commentary: Vignette 14.4

Nurses should never be physically abused at work. No other workplace considers violence "just part of the role," and nursing needs to ditch this unsupportive and dangerous attitude immediately. If a nurse feels physically threatened in a clinical situation, security needs to be called, and they need to take the problem seriously and be prepared to act. Nurses have been seriously injured and even killed at work. Being hurt is not part of getting an RN license. Period.

The issue of patients taking their frustrations out on nurses is also longstanding and needs to stop. In the kind of situation described, waiting rooms need to be as pleasant as possible, members and staff members need to be polite and professional. Patients need to be clearly told how long their wait may be and why they have to wait. A prominent complaint box along with clear evidence that the complaints are listened to and acted upon could also help diffuse patients' feelings of powerlessness and make nurses less likely to bear the brunt of their dissatisfaction. Also, managers need to make themselves available to hear patients' complaints and respond. Sometimes people just want to be heard, and the manager can fill that role better than an overworked staff nurse in a busy ED.

–Theresa Brown

Sabrina is actually identifying multiple issues. The first is the straightforward inappropriate behavior of a patient. The patient's behavior, however, is likely a symptom of a bigger organizational issue of inertia. This organizational ambivalence is displayed by the blanket acceptance of negative conditions such as the waiting-room environment, patient wait times, and patient abuse. This organization seems to have conditioned workers to accept these factors rather than empowering them to improve the conditions. Sabrina's nurse manager's response to her complaints reflects this serious organizational dysfunction.

It is unclear whether the dysfunction is based in the emergency department and associated management or if it extends to higher levels of the institution.

Sabrina is correct that it's unacceptable for patients to be physically aggressive toward nurses, and it is understandable that she is frustrated and scared. Sabrina's manager is also correct that this kind of behavior will occur from time to time. Nonetheless, the manager made three mistakes:

- She failed to validate Sabrina's concerns and instead told Sabrina to accept the status quo.

- She failed to examine the factors leading to the patient's actions.

- She failed to examine the organizational factors that led the patient's anxiety to escalate to such an extent.

A critical role of a nurse manager is to support nurses in ways that enable them to grow in confidence and professional excellence. The manager failed Sabrina here.

The patient in this example may have been terrified that he was having a heart attack and was being dismissed by the ED staff. It is possible that a few minutes listening to the patient, validating his fear and pain, and explaining how they determined it was not a heart attack may have prevented him from touching Sabrina at all. The behavior seems to stem from complete frustration that he was not heard and fear he was being dismissed in a potentially life-threatening situation.

There are ways to positively affect the ED environment and to model appropriate patient interaction. Nurses need training and support to quickly identify and problem-solve escalating patient anxiety and aggression. Certainly, decreasing patient anxiety is a worthy goal with many positive outcomes in any circumstance, and such training could be helpful across the board. Even in the case of patients who are aggressive because of altered mental status, training and support of nurses to manage and provide care is essential. There are countless strategies and models for dealing with these issues, but "just accepting it" is not one of them.

Sabrina could approach the manager with suggestions for training and programming. It is possible she may be more receptive to this focus on the functioning of the unit and all of the ED nurses rather than on a single personal incident. However, history indicates this may not be the case, and it may be an issue that needs to be taken up the organizational ladder.

–Kelly Dineen

Reflection

Is the culture at your hospital one that allows nurses to be taken advantage of or even abused? What measures can you and other nurse managers take to change the way your staff is treated?

Have nurses in your unit ever had experiences like the one described by Sabrina? Is this a typical occurrence, or something that happens only once in a while? What training could you provide nurses so that when such incidents do happen, they are prepared?

Vignette 14.5: Challenging Patients

On Shelly's psych floor, patents who are "difficult" often end up getting medicated by Natalie, the evening shift nurse. Since the hospital has a no-restraint policy, there's a protocol they follow when a patient seems to be escalating and possibly becoming aggressive. Natalie has a problem with adolescent boys, perhaps because her own sons have been a great challenge during their maturing years. If she has any grounds to medicate young male patients at all, she will, even if it violates protocol.

Last night at work, Joel, a 16-year-old admitted for depression, got agitated after his parents visited. This had happened the day before, and he was able to settle down and stop screaming with some redirection. As his nurse, Shelly assessed the situation and decided that talking to him one-on-one was appropriate. Before she could even say a word to him, however, Natalie appeared with meds.

"He's disrupting the unit and upsetting other patients," Natalie told Shelly. Natalie then informed Joel that if he wouldn't take a pill, she would have to give him an injection. Later, Shelly told Natalie it was upsetting to have her plan pre-empted by Natalie and asked if she had any insights into why she was quick to medicate. Of course, Natalie told Shelly that she was in the wrong, and the behavior continued.

Expert Commentary: Vignette 14.5

This is a troubling example, but it has a fairly straightforward solution from a management perspective. Presumably, the protocols in use on the floor were carefully designed and have been deemed appropriate by the clinical staff. If Natalie's use of chemical restraints violates the floor's protocol, then that behavior can be clearly addressed with her and the steps of the protocol can be reviewed.

Ideally, the nurse manager would probe further and find out why Natalie feels so strongly about medicating certain patients. If she is reacting to patients based on her own experience as a parent, a referral to employee assistance could be helpful. The entire tone of the manager's conversation can focus on, "I want to help you be the best nurse you can be," and not in any way punitive.

–Theresa Brown

Natalie's behavior is unacceptable, and she needs corrective action. In fact, she may need to be removed from the floor. She is not working in collaboration with her peers, nor is she in compliance with hospital guidelines or principles of nursing ethics. Not only is she verbally bullying other nurses such as Shelly, but she is literally intervening in patient care. This is abhorrent behavior in any setting, but is especially disturbing in the psychiatric setting, in which building trust and a sense of stability with the patient is paramount.

Natalie is overriding the better nursing judgment of her peers, restraining patients against hospital policy, creating a restrictive environment for the patients, and threatening patients into taking medication (the antithesis of consent).

Shelly approached Natalie in an appropriate and assertive way, expressing her feelings and concerns. Natalie is obviously having trouble accepting responsibility for her actions, and her own personal circumstances are probably clouding her judgment. Natalie needs professional help to identify her own biases, motivations, and distorted thinking and to isolate those from her behavior with patients.

If Natalie is to remain in her position, she also needs additional training and other remediation strategies to bring her nursing care into compliance with acceptable practices. She must receive training and support to mend her damaged relationships with peers and move forward in a collaborative manner. Her care should be mentored or monitored for some time during this process so as to not put patients in danger.

If there is a significant history here, or if previous attempts at remediation have failed, Natalie may need to be terminated. Allowing subpar nurses to continue in any position is harmful to the nurse, dangerous for patients, detrimental to the reputation of the unit and institution, and injurious to the professional reputation of nurses as a whole.

–Kelly Dineen

Reflection

Is the caseload on your unit full of challenging or "difficult" patients that take extra energy to care for? How can you help your staff to avoid "burnout" or "snapping out"?

When there is friction between two staff members or conflict over how to care for a patient, do you intervene, even when your help is not solicited?

Vignette 14.6: Stereotypes/Biases Against Patients

I worked in a small, rural hospital primarily staffed with nurses who had devoted many years of service to the institution. One morning during a shift report, when I was a new nurse and had been in the RN position for less than 8 months, we learned we had a patient with a diagnosis of HIV. One of the nurses boldly stood up during report and vehemently announced that she would not take care of this patient because of the HIV. She proceeded to inform us that he did not deserve our care and should be left to suffer. This was to be his punishment for his chosen lifestyle.

I sat stunned. This was a seasoned nurse who considered herself a mentor and nursing leader on the unit and within the facility. Those of us sitting in report looked at each other as she stomped out of the room muttering to herself about how nobody could make her take this person as a patient. This set a toxic tone for the beginning of our 12-hour shift together.

The staff working that day did not speak to that particular nurse the entire shift. I spoke up to volunteer and asked to have the patient as part of my workload for that day and for the next 2 days that I worked. As a new nurse, I could not understand how you could be a nurse for so many years and voice such a blatant bias against someone who desperately needed our care.

As this was a small hospital, my worry that the patient would learn of the scene that had played out that morning became a reality. I never knew how, but the patient did hear the story of the morning report. After hearing the story, the patient both thanked me and apologized to me for being there and needing my help. I did not have words to explain the behavior of the medical professional that morning. I told the patient I was glad to be able to help, and there was no apology needed.

The art and science of nursing enhance the holistic care we as nurses provide to our patients. We must be careful not to impose our own beliefs onto our patients through the care we give. I am extremely proud to be a nurse and would go to great lengths to never intentionally hurt a patient with my own words as that nurse did that day. This made a huge impact on me as a new nurse, and I have never forgotten the incident or the detrimental environment that was created and felt that day.

–Anonymous

Expert Commentary: Vignette 14.6

This story is both very understandable from a human perspective and unacceptable in terms of nursing practice. The older nurse was obviously way out of line, but her behavior resulted from ignorance of the science of HIV transmission and a moral prejudice against patients with HIV.

Hearing of this incident, the manager could act immediately to tell the entire staff that taking care of patients with HIV poses unique challenges, but no one is allowed to discuss such patients as undeserving of care. It also needed to be made very clear that the patient would never hear of the experienced nurse's comments, because inevitably it would make the patient feel less than human.

–Theresa Brown

This example illustrates that nurses as a group are people with their own biases and prejudices, just like the general population. It again illustrates the importance of separating feelings and judgments from professional behavior. In health care, the stakes of malfeasance based in deeply held negative judgments about patients are incredibly high. Nurses have to consciously work to be aware or mindful of these biases and how they could detrimentally affect patient care.

Certainly, the nurse in question approached her feelings about individuals with HIV in an incredibly negative manner. This could not have been the first time she examined her feelings about individuals with HIV. As a caregiver, she had an obligation to sort through these issues and her approach before such a patient appeared on her floor.

Her coworkers did not talk to her that day; in this case, an informal approach to group influence occurred through "shaming." Yet, she must have some degree of informal power over the group, because no one challenged her directly. It is somewhat surprising that no one was willing to engage her on her beliefs, how they might be based on mistaken knowledge, or why she could not separate her disapproval of certain behaviors from her disdain for the patient.

Like many nurses in the vignettes in this chapter, the nurse described here has lost her way. This does not mean that her peers need to tolerate inappropriate behavior. Indeed, they can support her as a person while clearly rejecting her behavior. Yet, this may be even more difficult to do in a hospital in a small, rural area because these nurses will be hard pressed to avoid each other professionally or personally if the relationship ends badly. It is even more important that the manager support their efforts to establish an appropriate group dialogue about this incident and potential similar incidents. In the absence of such action, this nurse has just established a precedent and a model for behavior that will be tolerated. In fact, if not already in place, this is the time to develop policies about patient coverage and the narrow criteria under which a nurse can request to not care for a patient. It is also a time to provide some condition-specific education on everything from transmission to appropriate care plans.

The manager must also work with this nurse individually and must require self-examination and behavior change. As a mentor in the group, this nurse has damaged her credibility in a very serious way. She must acknowledge her error and work to repair the damage. In the event the nurse is resistant to such efforts, the manager will need to have a serious discussion with her about her ability to remain in nursing in general and on the unit in particular. The manager must work to ensure actual change has occurred rather than just an "agreement" to take care of patients with HIV, because the nurse's biases will likely negatively affect care in the absence of real attitude change.

–Kelly Dineen

Reflection

Everybody has biases. What are yours? Be honest! Once you name them, you can work toward managing them. But until you face your own biases, it's unlikely that you'll be able to help your employees face theirs.

Have you noticed that any of your nurses exhibit biases against certain types of patients? Should a nurse with a bias be permitted to avoid caring for patients he or she finds objectionable?

Summary

Within every hospital, the emotional climate for both patients and nurses varies from floor to floor. Consider the newborn nursery, where the outcomes are almost always happy ones: Nurses smile and appear to enjoy their work. On the other hand, the operating room and other intensive care units seem to subsist on stress. In situations where high stress and turnover aren't balanced by teamwork and mutual respect, the culture is one of misery.

That culture doesn't change in one day, with one workshop, or with one book. Often, it doesn't change with just one person, but you may be the type of inspiring leader who can transform the workplace from stressed to blessed. Finding a few champions to work with you on resolving the obstacles that prevent nurses from being satisfied with the job they perform on your unit can be another option, as is implementing an orientation program that spells out behavioral expectations.

The satisfaction of your staff can be connected to the well-being and recovery of the patients you care for. This can be a great motivator, since the one thing nurses all agree about is their focus on helping patients!

Activity

Answer yes or no for the following scenarios. Is there ever a circumstance when it is acceptable for a nurse to:

- Speak harshly to a patient

- Withhold medication

- Be rough with a patient

- Speak negatively about patients

- Be rude to the patient's family

Have your staff members share their thoughts on these questions, and see if you can identify a minimum threshold for treating your patients with respect (especially difficult ones).

15 | on the battlefield: nurses under attack

Nurses experience different kinds of violence in the workplace. First, there are patients who act aggressively. To understand this situation better, Tema, Poggenpoel, and Myburgh (2011) interviewed nurses who had experienced violence from patients. Their participants reported feeling fear in the workplace, adverse physical and emotional symptoms, and use of cigarettes and other unhealthy substances for coping. These nurses worked on a psychiatric floor, which is one of the leading units where violence can occur.

In situations where aggression is a constant possibility, nurses described needing to be able to count on their colleagues to "have my back." Personal difficulties between nurses could sometimes interfere with the kind of teamwork needed to ensure safety.

Another source of violence is from coworkers, be they nurses or support staff. Our readings suggested that many nurses had witnessed subtle forms of physical aggression at the workplace. Bumping, elbowing, shoving, etc. were all used to convey anger and conflict.

Commentator Isabelle St-Pierre shares her expertise on this topic:

> As part of my doctoral work, I interviewed 19 nursing managers to specifically explore how they dealt with

intraprofessional aggression. While they all agreed that they had a huge role to play in positively responding to this ongoing and pervasive issue, they also verbalized how difficult it was for them to manage instances of peer-to-peer aggression.

[Nurse managers] identified several causes to explain the challenges they faced, such as (1) the extent of the problem (or just how common it was for nurses to abuse one another); (2) the propensity for staff to "informally" report instances of peer aggression while refusing to allow the manager to use their names when confronting the said perpetrator; (3) staff not really wanting to be involved in contributing solutions to the issue; (4) managers' limited visibility on the unit(s) related to their large span of control and heavy workload; (5) managers' personal ability and state of mind when dealing with aggression (some reported that they themselves were the victim of workplace aggression); and (6) the support managers receive when responding to instances of aggression (are they able to discipline employees and follow up with consequences, or are their disciplinary actions overturned?).

Sometimes, nurses report that coworkers are too friendly in a physical way, leading them to feel as if their boundaries have been violated. Hugging, patting, and rubbing may be well-intended gestures, but unless the recipient invites such behavior, it's best to stay hands off. Nurses described feeling uncomfortable with such physicality, even when it involved a nurse and her patients. Given the current raising of consciousness around the act of touching another person in the professional arena, nurse managers are well advised to model and encourage a "hands-off" environment.

According to an American Association of Critical-Care Nurses (AACN) position paper on workplace violence prevention, health care workers face the highest rate of violence of any industry, with nurses being three times more likely than other workers to be the recipient of aggression at the workplace. It's

not surprising that physical conflict—and conflict in general—
have been linked to poorer patient outcomes, but there are ways
to prevent these incidents.

AACN suggests that nurse managers need to do the
following:

- Develop prevention programs that involve both staff
  and administration.

- Establish clear policies that spell out expected behaviors as well as remediation for violent behaviors.

- Institute a confidential reporting procedure.

- Train employees.

- Follow up on incidents.

The American Nurses Association (ANA) also addresses the
issue of workplace violence (ANA, 2012). While there is no federal standard that addresses aggression, the ANA points out that
The Joint Commission passed standards mandating measures to
foster safety in the workplace. This gives nurse managers a new
kind of clout when advocating for safety in the workplace.

Another scenario involving physical aggression relates to
whistle-blowers. Casserly (2012) writes about this situation
in her article "When Snitches Get Stitches," published in her
column for businesswomen in *Forbes Magazine*. She found out
that physical aggression against people who report misconduct
(whistle-blowers) escalated from 4% in 2009 to 25% in 2011,
and that fists and staplers are the most common ways in which
violence is delivered.

Sometimes, the retaliation involves destruction of property.
Casserly believes the weakened economy has escalated anxiety
among workers to the point that expression of anger is more
extreme. This could certainly be true in a health care environment, where more is expected in less time, and fewer workers
must do what used to be the work of many.

Regardless of the source of physical aggression in the workplace, nurse managers have the task of ending such behaviors

quickly and definitively. Patients who are physically abused by nurses must be able to report such actions knowing that prompt measures will be taken to address the nurse aggressor. Certainly, nurses who are accused of being abusive of patients must be removed from direct care and appropriate actions taken to both investigate and remediate. Specific penalties vary from state to state, but the nurse manager must ensure that the issues are addressed.

If patients assault nurses, many institutions now permit nurses to press charges through the legal system, which means police officers are called to come to the scene of the violence. This practice is controversial, especially in psychiatric units where, many nurses believe, the possibility of aggression from a mentally ill patient is constant.

The National Advisory Council on Nurse Education and Practice (NACNEP; 2007) reports that in many states, assault of a nurse by a patient is not considered a felony, while in other states, assault by a patient on a physician is considered a felony and assault by a patient on a nurse a misdemeanor. Criminal considerations aside, NACNEP takes a strong stand on addressing workplace violence, which has a direct impact on nurse recruitment and retention.

NACNEP encourages prevention of assaults through the following:

- Adoption of standards of violence with legislative clout—i.e., in accordance with regulations from the Occupational Safety and Health Administration

- Education for nurses on prevention of and early intervention for violent behaviors

- Formal dialogue between nurses and administration about workplace safety to make sure there is a mutual agreement on addressing violence. Concern that reporting assaults will reflect poorly on their clinical abilities should not be a barrier for nurses.

- Collection of accurate data on violence against nurses, which can be used to develop best practices for prevention.

- Provision of adequate staffing and working conditions so that risk factors are reduced, especially in mental-health, emergency-department, and intensive-care units.

While a nurse manager may be inclined to minimize violence in an attempt to advocate for patients and achieve outcome measures established for his or her unit, employee safety is paramount. Violence-prevention programs for nurse managers must be implemented, and collaboration among all levels of administration and the institution's risk managers must occur to ensure that nurses can carry out their professional responsibilities in a safe and effective manner.

Vignettes, Commentaries, and Reflective Thinking

The remainder of this chapter presents vignettes about violence in the workplace, commentaries about the experiences represented in the vignettes, and opportunities to explore or reflect on the material.

Vignette 15.1: Physical Attack

Tara, a CNA on a pediatrics floor, is very aggressive physically. If she's on her way to provide patient care and someone else is in the hallway, she'll bump against them or somehow manage to have physical contact that borders on rough. Janet has never seen Tara act aggressively toward the kids they care for, but today Tara actually pushed Janet out of her way when she wanted to get in the lounge for her lunch break.

Janet feels like she is the only person Tara targets for this kind of behavior, and doesn't know what to do about it. Janet tells a friend, "I'm fairly new to the pediatrics unit, and don't want to create problems, but Tara bothers me and makes me wonder what will happen next. I don't feel safe with her around."

Expert Commentary: Vignette 15.1

As nurse managers, it is imperative that we create a safe environment for all of our staff. The statement by Janet is very disconcerting, and her concerns must be addressed. Nurse managers must create an environment in which staff members are not afraid to speak up regarding concerns in behavior, patient safety, and patient care. Hopefully, Janet's friend would encourage her to report this concern, and the response she receives from her leadership team needs to be supportive.

The nurse manager and Janet need to discuss the interactions with Tara. It is the responsibility of the unit leadership to address or help staff to address conflicts and behavioral issues at the unit level—hopefully in an informal manner first. It would be important to identify whether, in fact, Tara only behaves this way toward Janet, or whether it is her normal behavior. That may be hard to ascertain without having conversations with other staff or looking for opportunities for all of the leadership team to observe Tara's behavior.

If the situation is only between Tara and Janet, then a peer-to-peer conversation may be the best approach—but facilitated by a member of the leadership team. If Tara does behave this way with many staff, then the situation may require that leadership get involved in the conversation with Tara.

In any of the conversations, Tara needs to understand how her behavior is affecting her coworkers. It would be important to provide her with positive intent first, such as "We all want to work as a team in a healthy, pleasant environment." Feedback should focus on the specific behavior, not the person, and the impact that the behavior has on her coworkers. Tara needs to have the opportunity to respond and then discuss solutions.

If Tara is not open to peer feedback, leadership conversation, or changing her behavior, then nursing leadership may need to move to the disciplinary path. Physical abuse cannot be tolerated in the work environment. As nurse leaders, we need to set an appropriate example and be prepared to address these types of issues. Peer-to-peer accountability is a much more effective approach. Perhaps even Janet's friend could help Janet to speak with Tara.

—Lori Bechtel

Everyone establishes boundaries for touch and personal contact differently. Some nurses may be more touchy/feely, while others hold back and are reserved. The same is true for support staff. But given the imbalance of power between a nurse and a CNA, the nurse manager would have to wonder if Tara is using body language to convey a message she hesitates to speak. As nurse manager, I would act swiftly to determine whether this might be the case.

If Tara is just a more physical person and used to elbowing, patting, and jostling everyone, this is the time to raise her awareness about treating coworkers with the same guidelines she uses with patients—assuming there are no issues there. It's important for everyone to feel safe when they come to the unit.

Tara may not even realize she's being so physical. This is an opportunity to educate and reinforce "appropriate touch" to everyone and can be accomplished with an activity that asks staff to take a few minutes and give thumbs up or thumbs down to various forms of physicality. You might be surprised by how many people do or do not feel comfortable with an uninvited hug!

—Cheryl Dellasega

Reflection

The size of your personal bubble—the space into which you're not comfortable with others intruding—may be smaller or larger than those around you. Do you think your bubble is bigger or smaller than average? How does it make you feel when someone is in your bubble? Should the size of the bubble get bigger when you step through the doors to work?

Physical aggression is more than simply being inside someone else's bubble. Would you describe any of the nurses on your unit as physically aggressive, like Tara? What behaviors, in particular, do you think cross the line? As a nurse manager, what can you do to address this situation?

Vignette 15.2: Too Touchy

I currently work for a long-term acute care facility as a staff nurse and relief charge nurse. When I was given the chance to fill in for my chief nursing officer for a week, I jumped at the opportunity!

Acting in this role included being on call for the facility 24 hours a day. One night, I received a call about an incident at the facility involving the charge nurse and one of the staff nurses. The charge nurse stated that she had approached a staff nurse to give report. The staff nurse had previously stated that she "did not liked to be touched." However, the charge nurse approached the staff nurse from behind, placed her hand on the staff nurse's shoulder, and called her name to get her attention. The staff nurse became immediately angered by the touch of the charge nurse and shouted for the charge nurse not to touch her. The charge nurse apologized, but did not remove her hand. The staff nurse grabbed the charge nurse's hand and aggressively pushed it off her shoulder, resulting in a scratch on the charge nurse's hand.

I feel the shouting that occurred on the unit was unprofessional, and the charge nurse, being in a position of management, should have known how to diffuse the situation instead of allowing tension into the work environment. Patients and families were startled and on edge. The staff was also on edge, making it difficult to redistribute the patient assignments. I sincerely hope this doesn't occur in other professions. I understand that the staff nurse may have personal issues, but I think her reaction could have been handled better. It just seemed juvenile and unprofessional.

–Anonymous

Expert Commentary: Vignette 15.2

As a nurse leader, the situations that sometimes occur are hard to fathom. Sometimes, the first step may be to take a step back and think through our own feelings. Objectivity is sometimes difficult, because we all bring our personal feelings and reactions to situations. At face value, the present case seems to reflect an overreaction by the staff nurse to being touched. It would be important to find out why she reacted so vehemently. If there is an underlying reason for this response, most facilities have access to employee-assistance programs that may be helpful for this staff nurse. Personal space is very important to some people, and that should be respected in a work environment.

In addition, it would be important to find out whether the charge nurse was aware of the staff nurse's feelings about being touched and why she did not remove her hand when asked. There is a higher level of accountability that is expected of charge nurses, but sometimes they are simply staff nurses who are serving in that role for that shift. Although it would be beneficial, not all charge nurses are given the opportunity for training in managing difficult encounters.

In general, most organizations have some type of personal behavior and communication policy that nurse leaders can rely on for disciplinary action if needed. These types of policies address topics such as being open-minded and listening to other points of view, common courtesy, handling disagreements in a private location, respecting cultural differences, and working together professionally. Any behavior that could be considered intimidating, hostile, or harassing in nature such as yelling, invasion of personal space, touching, name-calling, or any communication that could be perceived as derogatory or discriminatory is not tolerated. These policies outline the possible courses of action for any employee.

The best method for handling physical-type negative behavior is constructively, with both parties involved, in a timely manner. It is imperative that these conversations are held face to face in a setting that is nonconfrontational for all involved and at an appropriate time. Email is not an option when discussing these types of incidents. Often, staff members do not grasp the implications of their behaviors. In fact, they may not even realize they are doing them. As nurse leaders, it is important to remain unbiased in our investigations into incidents such as this one and try to understand the perceptions of all parties involved. It is important not only to look for reasons for behaviors, but also to emphasize behaviors that will not be tolerated in a healthy work environment.

—Lori Bechtel

Nurses aren't the only ones who report issues with being touched physically, but given the intimate nature of our work, it might be assumed that we don't mind being tapped on the shoulder or patted on the hand. As a primarily female profession, nurses may take liberties with each other that wouldn't occur in a less homogenous workplace. (I think of the physicality of players on a football team; most likely, they wouldn't high-five and slap each other on the back in other circumstances.)

This doesn't mean it's right or automatically acceptable to touch a coworker. If the staff nurse had asked not to be touched, it's curious that the nurse in charge would not only do so but refuse to remove her hand when asked.

As a nurse manager, being respectful of coworker requests about the workplace whenever possible is part of your role—and a standard you set for others. Asking not to be touched is not an unreasonable request; indeed, individuals who have been abused or mistreated in the past may logically feel this way.

This situation needs to be addressed quickly so both the staff nurse and the charge nurse do not escalate into further aggression. As a trio, the three of you need to determine why each person acted as she did and what might make the situation better. Most likely, the charge nurse did not know about the "no touch" request and meant no harm by her actions—although she did persist when asked not to. The staff nurse was understandably upset by the charge nurse failing to honor her wishes, but she also responded roughly—although most likely without intention to harm. An apology, forgiveness, an expression of regret, and an expression of the intention to do better in the future, as well as other forms of restorative justice, can help both nurses move forward, but undoing the harm of the past will take continued effort and time.

—Cheryl Dellasega

Reflection

Physicality is very unique. Some people don't mind an impromptu hug or pat, while others consider such behavior offensive. How do you feel when other people touch you without you prompting the touch?

When you're at work, is the standard for touching tighter or looser? Can you imagine a scenario where touching—even innocent, well-intended touching—could make you uncomfortable? How would you respond? What, if any, obligation do you as the nurse manager have to try to make everyone comfortable?

Summary

A nurse we know is pregnant. It's her first child, and she's 7 months along, and for many reasons—workplace violence among them—she chose to stop working for the last few months of her pregnancy. When we asked her to explain a bit more, she told us that on more than one occasion, a patient she was caring for accidentally hit her stomach—pretty hard. She lost her first pregnancy, so she's probably hypersensitive to these things. But still, it's a tragedy that she felt like she needed to stop working in order to keep her baby safe.

Nurses may have their own issues, ranging from not wanting any uninvited touch due to a history of abuse, to adoring a spontaneous hug because that's how their family of origin interacted. Being sensitive to everyone's position on that continuum is a challenge, especially in a profession where your clients (patients) may feel it's ok to grab, kiss, or raise their voices to you.

Of course, violence is bad simply because it's violence. But there are also other consequences: Workplace violence can lead to feelings of fear, adverse physical and emotional symptoms, and negative coping mechanisms. Increasingly, young women see violence as an acceptable way to express emotion. At an interdisciplinary leadership conference for undergraduates a few years ago, one nursing student volunteered that she had punched a roommate during a disagreement. Her admission wasn't what shocked—it was her nonchalance about the incident.

Nursing is physical work. Nurses get bumped, pushed, prodded, and hit—and hopefully the *vast* majority of it is accidential or simply the result of a miscommunication. When it's not accidental, something is seriously wrong, and immediate steps need to be taken to try to resolve the issue. There is enough *unavoidable* workplace violence (e.g., the patient accidentially flails an arm against your face) that we absolutely cannot be adding to it with *avoidable* workplace violence.

Activity

People often assume that nurses won't mind being spoken to or physically touched in ways that would not be appropriate outside the hospital. One aspect of this is the personal bubble. Consider starting an awareness-raising campaign about the bubble, which is the space around you that you feel uncomfortable having people enter. (There are several online resources about the personal space bubble [PSB], including a post at needlemeethaystack.com/2010/02/08/bubble-pop/). Get volunteers to put up some info or share nuggets of information about the PSB. Examples of thought-provoking questions include the following:

- How big is your space bubble?
- Does your space bubble change depending on who you're talking to?
- Do you think the size of the bubble is cultural?
- What do you do when someone is inside your bubble?

- Are patients allowed to intrude into your space bubble because you're their nurse?

As a manager, it's really important to let your employees know that you support them with respect to inappropriate touch. Let staff members know that you're ready to back them up if anyone—patient or coworker—intrudes in their bubble in an unacceptable way.

16 | toxic culture/ environment

Most nurses are probably familiar with the frustrations that come with trying to implement new ideas, the glacial pace of change, and the cynicism of fellow employees about the effectiveness and trustworthiness of the organization. This cynicism has been labeled "organizational cynicism" (OC), and is known to be theoretically and empirically distinct from personality traits, including trait cynicism, negative affectivity, and skepticism (Rubin, Dierdorff, Bommer, & Baldwin, 2009). Organizational cynicism is only recently beginning to be studied in a health care setting; understanding the consequences of OC in this setting has the potential to be a powerful tool.

Organizational cynicism is defined as "an attitude resulting from a critical appraisal of the motives, actions, and values of one's employing organization" (Bedeian, 2007 p. 11). People who are organizationally cynical believe that the practices of their organizations betray a lack of principles such as fairness, honesty, and sincerity. This belief affects their affect, indicating that OC is felt as well as thought (Dean, Brandes, & Dharwadkar, 1998). OC is measured by asking people to indicate how much they agree with statements like the following (Wilkerson, Evans, & Davis, 2008):

- Any effort to make things better around here is unlikely to succeed.

- Suggestions on how to solve problems around here won't produce much real change.

- My company pulls its fair share of the weight in its relationships with its employees.

People who agree with the first two statements and disagree with the third statement are likely to be organizationally cynical. (If you want to explore your OC tendencies further, see Appendix C, "Organizational Cynicism Self-Assessment.")

The empirical study of OC is relatively new, so research on causes and effects is still in its infancy. However, research indicates that fewer opportunities for autonomous behavior predict OC, as do workplace hassles, psychological contract violations (the perception that the organization does not keep its promises), and procedural injustice violations (Luczwek, 2007; Naus, van Iterson, & Roe, 2007).

Recently, we conducted some research on OC in the medical center where we work. (Note that this study and the corresponding results are currently unpublished; data collection was completed about a year prior to this book being published.) We surveyed all the physicians and nurses who work in the hospital (n=2,835), with 47% of surveys returned (n=1,321). We found that the overall level of organizational cynicism was low (mean 2.7 on a 5-point scale, where 3 is neutral). We did learn, though, that nurses are more organizationally cynical than physicians (t=3.45, p<.01). Although we were not surprised to learn that nurses are more organizationally cynical than physicians, we were very surprised to discover that the overall level of OC was low. The reason we were surprised is because there seems to be a lot of anecdotal evidence that OC is a frequent problem in the health care setting. Indeed, whenever we tell anyone about our project, they have a story to tell about their own encounter with OC.

What these results may indicate (we need to do more data analysis to know for sure) is that most employees don't experience a whole lot of OC, but that a subset of the population experiences a high level of OC. For example, let's say that we surveyed 1,000 people and that the average response to the OC scale was 2.7, indicating a low overall level of OC. Let's assume further that we ranked those 1,000 people from lowest OC score to highest OC score. If we took the top quartile (which would be 250 people) and measured *their* average OC score, we strongly suspect that we would see a much higher number—perhaps 4 on a 5-point scale. In sum, our suspicion is that there exists a group of folks for whom OC is a serious problem, but, simultaneously, there is a group of folks who don't really experience OC at all. Although it's good that most employees don't seem to have a high level of OC, it only takes one or two cynical nurses to create a toxic work environment for an entire unit.

When employees experience OC, there are many negative consequences. These consequences can include negative behavioral work intentions, increased labor grievances in unionized organizations, decreased work motivation, and decreased extra-role behaviors (Kim, Bateman, Gilbreth, & Anderson, 2009). We also suspect (though we won't know for sure until we finish analyzing our data) that employees who are organizationally cynical have lower levels of institutional commitment and increased relational aggression.

Institutional commitment is a pretty big deal. In general, it is understood that there are three main types of institutional commitment (Allen & Meyer, 1996):

- **Affective commitment:** In this case, employees stay with the institution because of an emotional attachment to the organization. In other words, they stay because they like it. A person with high affective commitment would strongly agree with the statement "I really feel as if this organization's problems are my own."

- **Continuance commitment:** This is a "golden hand-cuffs" scenario. Employees stay with the institution because they feel like they have to. A person with high continuance commitment would strongly agree with the statement, "Right now, staying with my organization is a matter of necessity as much as desire."

- **Normative commitment:** These employees are with the institution because they feel obligated. A person with high normative commitment would strongly agree with the statement "I owe a great debt to my organization."

Discussion of organizational cynicism and institutional commitment may seem esoteric or even removed from the day-to-day practice of a nurse manager. But this literature gets at the heart of what it means to establish a positive culture and how that culture can influence worker morale. For example, decreasing levels of institutional commitment have been linked to health complaints among employees (Schalk, 2011).

So what are some things that nurse managers can do to try to improve their units' culture? From the perspective of organizational cynicism, there are at least two strategies that have been shown to be effective:

- **Include stakeholders in decision-making:** For example, when drafting a policy that primarily affects bedside nurses, be sure to have bedside nurses in the working group responsible for drafting the policy. And then—this is key—make sure folks *know* that one or more bedside nurses were involved.

- **Communicate change early and often:** One of the biggest predictors of OC is poor communication from leadership to employees. In a nearby hospital, two units were merged into one. The staff nurses in these two units were extremely frustrated because they felt that their perspective had not been adequately sought (see the preceding bullet), the change was passed down to them as a mandate from on high, and they didn't have as much advance notice as they would have liked.

To change the culture of a toxic workplace, Peggy Ann Berry says,

> *We have to acknowledge that most women have been so-cialized to be silent in mistreatment of self, to be shamed, blamed, and made guilty that bullying has occurred; or they have rationalized the behavior away, telling them-selves, "that's how she always is" (Dellasega, 2011; Fel-blinger, 2008). That has to stop. We can no longer be silent to the mistreatment toward each other or support staff, nor for the organizational bullying that occurs because of*

a culture that developed from the paternalistic, military hierarchy of hospitals, lack of job control, and blaming... But this also requires a choice of accountability for our own actions, for our own accountability to change at the peer level and push it up through that hierarchy and demand the cultural change of the organization for all employees.

Vignettes, Commentaries, and Reflective Thinking

The remainder of this chapter presents vignettes about toxic cultures and environments, commentaries about the experiences represented in the vignettes, and opportunities to explore or reflect on the material.

Vignette 16.1: Burned Out

In the summer of 2009, as a novice nurse educator, I went to a new institution to be the educator for the operating room. As I met the team leaders for each of the surgical services, I was introduced to two who had a history of being bullies.

The first team leader referred to me as the "damn nurse educator." When she saw me going toward the office, she would say, "Damn nurse educator, are you going to your toilet?" My office was previously a bathroom. This went on for about 3 months.

One morning, I gave an in-service with regard to a process change and requisition form for preparing patient specimens for the pathology department. As expected, the nursing staff had questions about completing the form. The second team leader was very much against the new process and stated the nurses should not be expected to do anything different from before. At the end of the meeting, she literally got in my face and screamed, "You are punishing the nurses!"

I reported these issues to both the director and associate clinical director of the OR. The associate clinical director asked me if any witnesses were present during the second team leader's rant. The director promised a meeting including himself, the team leader, me, and the associate clinical director, with a plan of disciplinary action. The meeting and disciplinary action never took place.

With regard to the first team leader, when I told the associate clinical director of her rude remarks, she looked shocked but didn't do anything. Months later, when it was decided that the first team leader needed to be put on a performance improvement measure due to her poor job performance, the associate clinical director became interested in her rude comments. She wanted to build a case against her and use all possible information.

I was shocked and angered by the behavior of these two nurses, as well as the passive attitudes of the directors in addressing the issues. I also noted that there were a number of staff who were aggressive and others who were passive-aggressive. While these behaviors can be found in any institution, it was more prevalent and acceptable in this operating room. It was a daily part of the culture.

After 3 months of working in the OR, I realized that the staff relied heavily on the support of their union representatives. In other words, it was very difficult to enact any kind of performance improvement or disciplinary action upon a staff member. It took a lot of time, mountains of paperwork, and volatile meetings with union representatives.

In the spring of 2011, I resigned my position and left the institution.

—Maxine L. Morris, MSN, BSN, RN, ACNS-BC, CNOR

Expert Commentary: Vignette 16.1

In this situation, the novice nurse educator is walking into a culture where bullying is tolerated, as evidenced by her knowledge of two team leaders' history at the time of her introduction to them. The question "Are you going to your toilet?" is a clear display of disrespect by the team leader. More importantly, from an organizational culture standpoint, she knows she is going to get away with it because of the implicit rules of behavior in this department. The director and associate clinical director of the OR are contributing to this disruptive behavior by using their leadership power to ignore it. No matter how assertive this new nurse is, it will be tough to set healthy limits while the leadership is basically saying that abusive language is OK.

Interestingly, the associate clinical director decides to take action later, with the goal of building a case against the team leader. Proactive opportunities to use examples of poor behavior to give constructive feedback, educate, coach, provide clear expectations, and encourage growth are lost. It seems a likely outcome that the team leader will eventually be terminated, and we know the nurse educator resigns, while little appears to be done to address the culture.

The costs of recruiting, hiring, and training replacement staff are probably much higher than organizational costs of finding ways to support management in addressing poor behavior; and, there is no guarantee that the same type of problem won't emerge all over again, because the underlying issues have not been addressed. Organizational support in the form of conflict management training for managers, giving and receiving constructive feedback for all staff, and increased administrative support are far more cost effective—and efficient—than dealing with a revolving door of new employees.

It is also worth noting that the in-service regarding preparing specimens raises questions about if, how, or when nurses on the front line are asked for input about process changes. If input is not sought, or is sought but not listened to, this would be an example of the culture not really respecting the nurses who do the work. When healthy channels for input don't exist, it is predictable human behavior to become passive-aggressive, aggressive, or passive in our expression. Key leadership skills for nurse managers include validating input and setting limits. In any case, the team leader yelling in the educator's face is inappropriate!

—Beth Boynton

I am going to speak both to the target and to management. For the target, failure to respond to the team leader's disrespectful name-calling the first time sets precedent for all further interactions between the team leader and "the damn nurse educator." The first interaction required push back to set the standard of her expected treatment by others. I can't guarantee it would work, but confrontation (cognitive rehearsal) with incivility and disrespect has been known to help new nurses communicate effectively the first time to this behavior (Griffin, 2004). Unfortunately, the inability to respond immediately to the bully is what makes the nurse educator a target for bullying. And, the team leader continued because she could get away with bullying behavior. The director and associate clinical director of the OR needed to respond immediately to the nurse educator concerns. Good nurses leave toxic cultures, even in this economic environment.

How does a manager prevent overboard reactions like the one by the second team leader? One way is to be present when changes are initiated. In addition, adults require context in learning a new system and the reasons why a change has occurred. Although the second team leader went overboard about the new system, she also required a calm response from the director or associate clinical director, to be asked why she thought it was punishment, and to be told why the change was occurring. As stated, bullies get away with it because they can. And the presence of the passive-aggressive and aggressive nurses that the nurse educator observed has a lot to do with the current management style.

In deciding how to respond to this particular situation, there are three broad choices:

- Take a deep breath, and remember that it is not personal. Maxine did nothing wrong to warrant any of this behavior.

- When addressing the issues with first-line management, Maxine could ask when the behavior will be addressed, either individually or in a group in-service.

- Maxine could inform first-line management that if the issue is not addressed, her next step is up to the next level, involving HR labor management, which deals with union issues.

There is little change in a toxic culture without change in leadership, either by education and determination or exit. The current management style seen, in which management does nothing until they have to, is a *laissez faire* style. Nothing is done (hands off) as long as the work gets done. If Maxine goes over first-line management, she will likely be pegged a whistle-blower for airing the "dirty laundry" on the cultural dynamics of the unit, keeping her a target or forcing her out by social exclusion by those she educates and those to whom she reports. She would have had to have a dose of healthy self-respect and self-care with social support outside work to survive the toxic culture. If the toxic culture can't change (remember, the whole facility can be toxic), Maxine made the only choice she could between her psychological health and that job.

—Peggy Ann Berry

Reflection

How DO you respond when the people on and off the job are passive-aggressive or just plain rude? Do you find it's more difficult to manage your feelings and responses when you seem to get that behavior from all sides?

What describes rude and incivil behavior at work? What might it say about the culture of your unit if your colleagues are chronically putting you and others down?

Culture can seem like an amorphous, intangible idea that is hard to wrap your arms around. How can you begin to get the pulse of your unit's culture? What steps will you take if you find that the culture is not what you want it to be? What are your obligations as the nurse manager?

Vignette 16.2: Ambitious Attributes

Cassie realized early on in nursing school that she wanted to become a midwife. Because all the programs she's considering require 2 years of experience in L&D, she obtained a job in L&D, even though she would have preferred to just go straight into a midwifery program.

Positions in L&D are very competitive, so the other new nurses were jealous when Cassie got the job. Cassie discovered that the nurses she works with aren't so supportive, either. Bobbi, a nurse who was the newest until Cassie arrived, asks her why she wants to work on L&D. Cassie replies truthfully, noting that she hopes to continue her education to become a midwife.

Bobbi's attitude toward Cassie changes completely. "I can see you won't be making any commitments to this job," she says. "The rest of us know we want to work here indefinitely, but you're just using us to get ahead."

Cassie tries to explain, "Maybe someday I will become one of the midwives who currently works so well with the nursing staff," but Bobbi gets even angrier.

"You should have told them you were only wanting to get experience so you could move on," Bobbi says and walks away. Cassie thinks to herself, "I was honest, not deceptive."

Expert Commentary: Vignette 16.2

What shines through loud and clear in this vignette is a lack of respect for self and others. Cassie is excited about her career path and shows initiative in creating opportunities while being willing to gain valuable experience that will contribute to her success. This seems admirable and is to some extent a reflection on the organization's willingness to support her and her honest intentions. This is a good thing!

On the other hand, where is all this jealousy and fear of being "used to get ahead" coming from? Ironically, even though assertiveness arises from a sense of self-esteem, it can be nurtured or thwarted by leadership and workplace culture. Despite indirect, tough-to-measure connections among self-esteem, speaking-up, and patient safety, it makes sense to look for organizational opportunities to positively influence them.

—Beth Boynton

One of the hardest things to do as a manager is to replace staff on a unit that is a stepping stone into advanced practice. With that, the unit has turnover. There are some nurses who enjoy giving nursing care without stepping into higher education and the advanced-practice role. However, there are those nurses who want an advanced-practice role. Nurses who stay in staff positions can grow resentful of the turnover and of training new nurses who will leave once they have gained enough of the required experience to enter into an NP or other program. Don't let your seasoned nurses become resentful toward the nurses who will leave the group to further their education.

As the manager of a stepping-stone unit, you can set the tone so staff members see turnover from advanced-practice entry as empowering the profession. You can also work with those you hire on the time frame for notice of resignation to ensure you'll be able to find a new hire with adequate orientation time before your new advocate for nursing leaves for school.

—Peggy Ann Berry

Reflection

Is your unit a "stepping stone" unit? How do you as a nurse manager balance commitment and career ambitions among your staff? Do you think the quality of care you deliver is better or worse because of it?

Is there an interpersonal divide between "long-haul" nurses and the ones who are just passing through? Do you contribute to the divide, and if so, how? What can you do to mitigate it?

Vignette 16.3: Organizationally Cynical Energy Vampires

Vicki works with Margo, a full-time RN on the orthopedic floor. Margo is talkative and tends to engage coworkers in conversations rather than comments. Most of her talk is negative and denigrating to the hospital in general and to the orthopedic unit in particular.

Vicki has found that she is starting to avoid Margo because she sucks her energy. Vicki talks to her coworkers about it, and they agree. Eventually, it gets bad enough that the unit nurses decide to take the issue higher. "It's exhausting to even listen," Tina, another nurse, tells the nurse manager. "That woman [Margo] is like an energy vampire. You can't break away from her!"

Vicki says, "I feel like Margo gets in the way of patient care, because she could keep you involved with her for valuable minutes."

The nurse manager knows what Tina and Vicki are saying is true. In fact, she also avoids having interactions with Margo, which does nothing to improve the situation.

Expert Commentary: Vignette 16.3

In the situation with Margo, everyone but she seems to know about her negative talking and energy drain. The respectful thing to do would be to give Margo direct feedback about how her behavior is perceived and affecting others. The nurse manager is avoiding giving the feedback and so are Margo's colleagues. Not only that, but the nurse manager allows Margo's colleagues to talk with her about it but does nothing. All of this is somewhat passive-aggressive and is a form of ganging up on Margo without her even knowing it.

This doesn't excuse Margo's behavior but helps to explain its pervasiveness. The nurse manager needs to address concerns with Margo and look at the organizational factors that contribute to all of the staff's behavior. The steps the nurse manager can take to turn this around include the following:

- Talking to Margo

- Encouraging colleagues to give Margo feedback

- The more long-term culture change of creating an environment where respectful feedback is the norm

To achieve this, the nurse manager must do the following:

- Acknowledge what is wrong with the current culture.

- Provide training in giving and receiving constructive feedback.

- Create practice and learning-curve opportunities for developing new behaviors.

- Coach struggling individuals.

- Eventually, discipline those not willing or able to communicate respectfully.

The nurse manager may also demonstrate assertiveness by asking her supervisor for some support in addressing these issues.

—Beth Boynton

As the manager, take a deep breath, remind yourself that it is not personal, and ask if Margo has any solutions that would stop the complaints. Make her feel safe with this exchange. She may have solutions; it's just everyone has gotten tired of listening to her. If there is no solution or basis for her complaints, tell her it must be so hard to work in a place she is so negative about. Let her know how ineffective and unproductive the complaining has become for everyone and that the negativity pushes away her peers.

Ask if she has a personal issue that is negatively affecting her life. Discuss a voluntary referral to an employee assistance program (EAP) to help her move beyond the cynicism and vent to the therapist only. Begin a coaching file to work on behavior and monitor the exchanges on the floor. If the initial talk and coaching do not stop the negative behavior, speak with HR about a mandatory referral to the EAP and how to progressively discipline. In addition, disciplinary action may be needed to drive the point that negativity will not be tolerated.

—Peggy Ann Berry

Reflection

Do you know anyone who is an "energy vampire"? Which of his or her behaviors are most bothersome? How do you handle these types of people?

Colleagues who sap energy can be exhausting to be around and difficult to avoid. Do you think there are any negative consequences to having someone like that on your staff? What might those consequences be? What can you do to try to change things for the better?

Vignette 16.4: Special

Krista is the nurse manager for a large urban ED. At the hospital where she works, ED nurses must have a year of experience and complete a special orientation program. At administrative meetings, Krista constantly asks for "special exceptions" and dismisses any complaints about the ED.

When the nursing supervisor announces a new-nurse recruitment program, Krista endorses it wholeheartedly. "I really need staff desperately," she says. "Make sure you find nurses with experience and an interest in emergency nursing."

The other nurse managers roll their eyes behind Krista's back. They complain about the "special treatment" Krista and her nurses receive and the different standards for the ED. "Nothing happened when I issued a complaint after one of the evening ED nurses cursed at one of my nurses during a transfer," Lynn comments. "They just told me, 'The ED is such a stressful place. You just have to understand how difficult it is.'"

Her nursing colleagues agree, sharing other stories of the favoritism shown to the ED and its staff.

Expert Commentary: Vignette 16.4

In this case, the lack of mutual respect is similar to that of Vignette 16.2, and many of the same organizational concerns and questions apply. All staff members deserve to be treated respectfully. Specific to this scenario is the stress involved in working in the ED and how that is or isn't addressed.

Rather than being an excuse for abusive behavior, the organization has an opportunity to consider how it can support its staff. Part of this requires setting respectful limits, having the staff delegate, and navigating potentially martyring behaviors. Nurse managers must be very clear that disruptive behavior such as cursing is never OK. The underlying message is, "If you can't behave respectfully toward your patients and colleagues, then you are not an effective ED nurse. If stress is influencing your behavior, let's talk about it and problem-solve together." If the organization isn't going to help problem-solve, stress and resentments will likely be buried deeper, and their impact on relationships will manifest in some way. The silos created with this us-versus-them mentality will take their toll on communication during handoffs; ultimately, patient safety will be at risk.

—Beth Boynton

The same standards should apply to all units in the hospital. To show favoritism to any one unit related to stress is not acceptable. It is chaos that needs to be controlled. There needs to be zero tolerance for aggressive overt or covert behaviors among staff nurses and units. If the culture is going to change, management needs to stop justifying the negative behaviors and start educating on how to work together as one system.

—Peggy Ann Berry

Reflection

Are all units created equally? Do you think that because units are different, they should be treated differently; or should they all be treated the same in order to promote fairness? Are certain units favored in your institution? Which ones? Why? What effect does this favoritism have on the other units in the organization? Does it affect morale?

Vignette 16.5: Unsupportive Support

Annabeth is new to the hospital where she currently works. It's different from other places she's worked in that the physicians are not normally on site. To get in touch with a physician, nurses are supposed to ask the unit clerk to page him or her.

One day, Annabeth has a patient with low blood pressure. She asks the unit clerk to page the physician, and the unit clerk does so. However, when the physician calls back, the unit clerk does not notify Annabeth that he is waiting on the line, so Annabeth misses the call.

Annabeth complains to a colleague, "It totally slowed up the process of patient care and added more stress to my day! I'm definitely getting the feeling that if I do anything to make the secretary's job harder, like ask her to page a doctor—which I'm pretty darn sure is one of the main components of her job—she makes *my* job harder. It just sucks that we can't support each other!"

Expert Commentary: Vignette 16.5

A unit clerk who does not notify a nurse that the physician is returning her call is a dangerous member of the team, and Annabeth's fears of retaliation are suggestive of underlying cultural issues. The nurse manager will need to clarify what happened and set clear expectations of communicating phone calls to nursing staff. Is there a possibility that a page was not heard, Annabeth was on break, or the process was unclear? If there are indeed underlying conflicts between these staff members, the nurse manager may need to intervene.

Maybe paging the doctors is a new part of the unit clerk's job. In situations where old habits exist and new efforts to change them are initiated, it is helpful to give employees the benefit of the doubt—once or twice. In the meantime, make new expectations very clear and if the unwanted behavior happens again, start to think about including disciplinary action as part of the process. Annabeth would also benefit from assertiveness training and coaching, which, of course, will be more effective if the underlying cultural issues are addressed. A process that "asks the unit clerk to page them" rather than "tells the unit clerk to page them, (with courtesy)" is a one-word change that makes the process much clearer!

—Beth Boynton

Annabeth needed to have a conversation with the unit clerk as soon as she was aware of the delay to understand whether this was done on purpose. If so, the manager needed to be pulled in immediately. This is a situation in which one person uses legitimate processes to undermine a nurse's ability to care for her patient, which could result in serious harm. The unit manager sets the expectations of the unit and enforces a zero-tolerance policy for this behavior, including how lapses in communication are handled. If this has been an ongoing issue, the manager needs to take action to stop it. One pivotal support staffer who power-plays with patient safety needs to be held accountable for her actions.

Each of us has to be accountable for our own behavior and not tolerate behavior that will affect patients and ourselves. However, the responsibility for setting the tone is squarely on the shoulders of leadership and management. When issues come up, leadership should act on it. I am not talking the knee-jerk reaction of firing perpetrators, however. This is a joint educational process with leadership and all employees. Leaders set the performance standards and the way staff members communicate with each other.

—Peggy Ann Berry

Reflection

How would you rate your support staff on being "supportive"? Navigating the hierarchy in medicine can be a challenge—not just between physicians and nurses but between nurses and folks like unit clerks. What strategies do you use for these types of challenges?

Are you a "flat-heirarchy" type of person (i.e., power is shared horizontally rather than vertically)? One helpful approach is to think that everyone is there to work as part of the team and deliver high-quality care to patients. But what do you do when one member doesn't seem to have the team's interests at heart?

Vignette 16.6: Replaceable

The North Henry Hospital is small, suburban, and a bit out-dated. Many of the nurses who work there have nowhere else close by to get a job. Morale is low.

"Why do doctors get a special lounge and not nurses?" Jama, an SICU nurse, asks.

"Who decided that we have to go through our supervisor before calling a physician for orders?" demands Melody, a NICU nurse.

"How can they expect us to work four 10-hour shifts that are really 12 hours?" asks Olivia, an ED nurse. "The doctors aren't expected to stay overtime!"

When these comments come to the attention of the director of nursing, she tells the charge nurses to dispel any complaints. The DON's advice is to tell "whiners" that "we all know nurses are lucky to even have a job here. Any one of you can be replaced with a day's notice."

Expert Commentary: Vignette 16.6

The tone for a toxic culture is set by the DON's advice to "whiners": "We all know nurses are lucky to even have a job here. Any one of you can be replaced with a day's notice." She may be getting the same message from her leaders, but it is an alarming one.

When leadership doesn't care what staff members at any level think or feel, they set the stage for unsafe communication, disengagement, and resentment. They may get compliance with rules and regulations in the short term, but the impact on the culture will be immeasurable damage in terms of communication, collaboration, morale, and safety.

Some of these nurses' concerns may be unreasonable or unrealistic, but finding ways to validate and to consider input will help develop a healthier workforce and workplace. Some of their concerns may warrant staffing or scheduling changes, team-building efforts, training in delegating, or a closer look at how staff nurses are spending their time. Respecting feedback means validating it, considering it, and possibly using it but not necessarily agreeing with it.

Notice how these statements differ in tone from the DON's and are empowering while maintaining clear leadership authority:

- "I can understand that a nurses' lounge would be appealing to you, Jama, but we do not have financial support for that right now. Perhaps we could be creative about other space in the hospital and build some inter-departmental spirit in the process. Would you like to talk with nurses on other units and HR and let me know any ideas you come up with?"

- "If your 10-hour shifts are turning into 12 hours, we need to take a close look at that. Let me know what's happening to keep you here longer, and we can brainstorm solutions. Can you meet with me today or tomorrow about this for 10 or 15 minutes? I'll check with other staff as well."

—Beth Boynton

The workforce and management are at odds with each other. Physicians are treated with respect, and nurses are treated like handmaidens to the hospital and the physicians. This hospital is ripe for a union, a sentinel event, and a lawsuit because administration does not consider these nurses valuable. Patient satisfaction is linked with nurse satisfaction; these nurses are not satisfied, however, and the hospital administration does not care.

As a manager of a unit, establish trust, protect your people, and treat them with respect. Encourage them to support each other on and off the job. Find ways to work around the administration's toxic attitude toward them. Require professional communication between staff and physicians and model it daily. Push up through that mess of an organization with evidence on treating employees as assets, not "throw-aways," and stress how a psychologically safe environment improves patient care.

—Peggy Ann Berry

Reflection

Do you feel valued or replacable in your position? How do members of your staff feel about their worth to you and the institution?

Vignette 16.7: Dirty Laundry

Hannah, a new nurse who is right out of an associate degree (AD) program, is openly critical of her coworkers. She questions why they use outdated procedures in the OR and points out the shortcomings of other nurses, whom she describes to her friends as "too slow, too old, or too fat."

One evening after a hectic day in the OR, Hannah logs on to her Facebook account and posts a negative comment about her coworkers. "These nurses are so lazy, they practically sleep on the job," she types.

One of the nurses has a teenager who recognizes Hannah as her mother's coworker and shares the comment. The next morning when Hannah arrives at work, her manager tells her she should look for another job, since she obviously can't be part of the "OR team."

Expert Commentary: Vignette 16.7

Hannah's communication with her coworkers is way out of line, and her social media outburst is a reasonable cause for termination. However, prevention factors that involve the organizational culture should also be considered in this scenario. What concerns might have come up during the interview process? What is the organizational expectation for interprofessional communication, and how is it made clear to staff? What happens during orientation to ensure that respectful communication is the norm? What is the nurse manager's role and skill level in addressing inappropriate behavior from the very beginning? Also, is Hannah's feedback about outdated procedures and sleeping on the job accurate? Despite Hannah's inappropriate manner of giving the feedback, such information should not be ignored.

In all the vignettes in this chapter, there are individual and organizational behaviors that contribute to unhealthy workplaces and outcomes. Nurse managers who seek to understand and address both can have an amazing impact on communication, teamwork, morale, patient experience, cost-effectiveness, and safety. Any facility that empowers its nurse-management team with training, practice, and coaching to give and receive constructive feedback will go a long way to ensuring its success in managing and leading teams, as well as developing effective peer relationships.

—Beth Boynton

If the laundry is that dirty, wash it! Hannah may be frustrated and angry for a reason or due to other issues going on. Rather than tell Hannah to look for another job, the manager should be questioning her on the details that caused this outburst. Yes, there are more appropriate ways of voicing disapproval up the chain of command, but Hannah may not have any other way of voicing her frustration. It could be that the manager's door has been closed to her voicing complaints. Or, the OR staff may be bullying Hannah and not working with her in the OR.

The manager also needs to discuss how to verbalize issues within the work area or to move them up through the chain of command. Hannah needs to learn to constructively communicate with her manager. At the same time, her manager needs to actively listen to Hannah.

—Peggy Ann Berry

Reflection

How do you manage the releationship between work and social media sites like Facebook? How do you decide which, if any, job-related thoughts and events are appropriate to post to your social media pages? Does your institution have a social media policy?

What are the deeper implications of Hannah's post? Hannah clearly doesn't feel like a member of the OR team. Who is responsible for that? The rest of the team members? Hannah? The nurse manager? Higher administration?

Summary

Organizational cynicism is a pretty big deal. When the culture of an organization is toxic—when employees believe that their organization is inefficient, unfair, dishonest, and insincere—there can be drastic consequences. In other settings, organizational cynicism has been shown to decrease the quality of employee performance. Some important questions for managers and administrators to consider are:

- What is the impact of organizational cynicism on the micro and macro levels?

- Does organizational cynicism on your unit lead to decreased employee performance?

- Could organizationally cynical nurses provide care that is harmful to patients (unintentionally, of course!).

The silver lining of organizational cynicism is that *it's a problem we can fix.* OC is caused by the leadership of an institution—and can be solved by the leadership of an institution. To reduce organizational cynicism, leaders should:

- Begin by naming the problem.

- Involve key stakeholders in idea brainstorming/ development.

- Communicate change early and often.

OC is often a result of employees feeling as though their voice is not heard or respected or that their work doesn't matter to the institution. If you—and other members of the leadership team—can successfully manage your institution's culture, you will have made a substantial contribution to the health and well-being of your patients. Plus—as an added bonus—you might discover that you start looking forward to going to work!

Activities

Sometimes, creating a physical change can lead to an attitude change. Talk to staff members and ask them to identify the number-one physical problem with the work environment. Is it too small? Too cluttered? Boring paint colors? Then, design a contest and have people submit ideas for how to address whatever was identified as the number-one problem. Have two or three people review the suggestions and identify the one that seems best. Then make it happen!

Alternatively, to increase awareness of and appreciation for the work of each team member, spend some time "shadowing" different employees and make a list of how how their actions influence patient care. For example, a nurse may spend extra time speaking with a family member, which will lead the patient to have a better visit. The unit clerk may go out of his or her way to put up holiday decorations that create a cheerful and festive mood. A physician you work with frequently may give an employee positive feedback that contributes to his or her professional self-worth.

17 | conclusions

Toxic nursing is a real threat to the nursing profession. It's not unusual for a nurse manager to be caught in the midst of mayhem that requires a skill set including patience, flexibility, creativity, and a bit of humor to resolve. When turmoil invades the workplace and leads to persistent negativity and friction, unhealthy and even harmful behaviors can become entrenched and normalized, creating a "culture of conflict." Don't wait for this to happen on your unit—be proactive in applying the information throughout this book to your unit. Remind yourself to be ABLE:

A= Act now to address conflict, relational aggression, and cynicism, rather than waiting until later.

B= Bolster your belief in all team members, and show that you believe they are talented, important, and appreciated by both you and the organization.

L= Lead through example. Show your staff that you are willing to use the same behaviors you expect from them, both on the unit and in interacting with other nurse managers and higher administration.

E= Expect excellence and empower your employees to achieve professional goals they set.

Keep in mind that some of the relational styles of nurses that lead to trouble seem to be patterns women in general have experienced for centuries. Historically—and perhaps still today—women were socialized to avoid overt conflict, to prioritize their roles as mother, wife, and daughter, and to focus on the "tend and befriend" approach. These roles and approaches can promote stress and challenge women in the workplace. Within the small community of a hospital, specialty, or unit, problems such as relational aggression and the conflict associated with it can sabotage even the best manager because of its pervasive nature.

Understanding the causes and complexity of chaos and crisis is an important first step. Our exploration of nursing narratives provided insight into some if not most of the situations real nurses find difficult.

For example, from the very beginning of employment, new nurses can be the subject of precepting gone bad, drama mamas, the local gossip grapevine, and cattiness as well as cliques. That doesn't mean newbies are blameless or helpless victims; they may come with baggage or an agenda that offends their coworkers from day one.

With varied educational pathways into nursing, respect for and tolerance of differences is crucial. The demand for nurses will continue to increase; as it does, innovative educational programs and alternative ways of learning will evolve. In the future, it is likely that there will be more difference than similarity in the educational backgrounds of any given unit of nurses.

Within a given workday, the potential for conflict and challenge is ever present, as multidisciplinary workers interact with each other and the people they are there to care for. Relationships between nurses and physicians and patients and families are challenged by technology, time, and tradition, but the minimum expectation is courtesy, respect, and safety.

In addition to problem behaviors, loyalty and longevity are influences in the health care workplace—in both good and bad ways. When nurses support nurses, incredible outcomes can occur. But when personal issues interfere with professional performance or relationships are strained by competition, the nurse manager may have to deal with negative fallout. As with many other professions, the boundaries between on- and off-the-job personas are blurring due to social media, changing standards, and a more fluid workforce.

Nurses who stand out may attract attention for unwanted reasons: gender, speaking in a foreign language, being at extreme ends of the age continuum (i.e., very young or very old, both defined differently than in the past), or having a certain status within the institution, to name a few. Any of these descriptors has the potential to create trouble unless the nurse manager can embrace, rather than stigmatize, diversity. Conflict that occurs around these situations in particular seems to be the catalyst for a nurse to declare, "This is illegal! I'm going to hire an attorney!"

While discrimination, harassment, and mistreatment used to be the purview of human resources or legal, they are now often addressed by the nurse manager. Dealing with these complex issues requires a combination of communication, motivation, and determination. At times, the manager must be a businessperson; at other times, the manager must be a listener or kindly parent; and at still other times, the nurse manager must be an expert conflict mediator. The ultimate challenge is to know the appropriate time to access which skill.

It's true that sometimes nurse managers are the source of strife. An inexperienced and ineffective leader is likely to be readily detected in the small community of a nursing unit, placing pressure on leaders to grow into their roles extraordinarily quickly. Being open and able to accept feedback about yourself and your work product can help a nurse manager become just such a leader.

If you're a new manager, one way to build relationships and simultaneously increase your management skills is to honestly seek the feedback of those you're managing. One of the authors of this book recently became the director of a program. She's pretty junior and was a little horrified at the prospect of directing some wonderfully skilled, exceptionally wise, and very senior colleagues. So she was honest. And she was *humble*. She frequently reminded them how much they had to teach her, but she also often reminded them what she was doing to make their jobs easier.

Within the larger system of hospital politics, nurse managers must often play middleman between administrators and staff. Juggling the need to carry out one's job in accordance with metrics or standards imposed by authorities while supporting the staff nurses who work to help produce measurable, quantifiable care can challenge even the most experienced nurse. Transparency is of great help in such circumstances, even when the manager lacks a definitive answer or is just as confused about the rationale for new policies and procedures as his or her staff.

Unfortunately, the outcome of toxic nursing can be hazardous to the health of both nurses and patients. Violence within the workplace is escalating in general, and for nurses who work in high-risk areas, fear for personal safety can be constant. At times, the staff nurse can become a patient when assaulted or mistreated. Caring for staff while caring for patients is the unique assignment of the nurse manager.

Two other topics need to be discussed: legal concerns and ethics. In our current litigious health care environment, the legality of workplace behavior and questions about the necessity of finding an attorney are all too frequent considerations. By way of example, this not-too-long-ago exchange occurred with a woman who sought to discuss her work situation.

"Rachel" had just taken a new position within the institution where she had worked for more than a decade. She was a hard worker and left one unit for another on good terms with her former boss.

The new manager was far less enthusiastic about Rachel's work product, however. As so often happens, the more pressure and tension that arose from the conflicted employee-employer relationship, the harder it was for Rachel to thrive.

As the manager pushed back against Rachel's questions about the status quo and requests for a more thorough orientation, the tension escalated. Rachel wondered about the possibility of a "harassment" or "hostile work environment" claim against her new boss.

Rachel was sure an attorney would take her case, because she had carefully copied correspondence from her manager and kept a detailed journal about the troublesome incidents she experienced at work. When she sought help from a friend who worked with several attorneys specializing in employment law, Rachel was shocked to learn she would almost certainly have to pay for more detailed legal advice.

She told her friend: "I think a lawyer will take my case for free, because it's worth a lot of money. Everyone tells me that's what I should do, and that I'll get a big settlement."

"Really? Would you work for free for a month?" her friend asked.

It's a difficult negotiation, but just as Rachel wouldn't come in and give her employer a week of free work, attorneys are not likely to invest time and energy without some initial payment for their service. In this scenario, although Rachel was disturbed and upset about her new job, the burden of proof in a lawsuit would be on her, not the manager. She would have to prove she was being harassed because of her age, gender, race, or a disability.

The emotional toll of taking this on while continuing to work for the person she was hoping to sue would be significant. Rachel's friend encouraged her to try to talk to her boss about the issues and then go on to human resources if needed.

About a month after their talk, Rachel ran into her friend. Rachel had just returned from vacation in the Caribbean and was happy to report she had transferred to a different position, with a manager who seemed pleased to have her. The situation was resolved without legal action, and Rachel found a happier place to work because she was talented and loyal.

The Rachel scenario has replayed many times in our interactions with nurses, leading us to read David Yamada's work on "therapeutic jurisprudence" (Yamada, 2008). Yamada, an attorney, encourages prevention of lawsuits whenever possible—"prevention is the cure"—and offers some general guidance that relates to both individuals and institutions. Although many of the specifics play out on a state-by-state basis, it's worth checking out his suggestions. Appendix D, "When It's Time to Get a Lawyer," also provides some excellent general advice from a different attorney on this topic.

Although a discussion of professional ethics was not explicit in any of the commentaries, carrying out the responsibilities of a registered nurse in is a part of civility and professionalism. Most of the vignettes describe unprofessional behavior within the work setting. As a nurse manager, you need to model not only professional but ethical behavior. Unfortunately, the line for this becomes increasingly blurred as social media plays a bigger and bigger role in our interactions. Some intriguing ethical considerations are:

> *Although nurses are committed to protecting privacy and confidentiality of information, when, if ever, is it acceptable to discuss issues such as a difficult patient or family member?*

> *When nurses feel their employers don't value their contributions or consider their well-being, how obligated are they to work overtime or give extra effort to improve patient care?*

> *If there is conflict on a unit, whose needs come first? Are nurses, the providers of professional care at the bedside, most important, or should the support staff and/or management take priority?*

> *Should a nurse present a particular professional appearance, or is it OK to have multiple piercings and tattoos that may be visible, even with a uniform?*

In these times of toxic nursing, nurse managers are the ones to take charge in a way that can change the culture of health care. Transformational leadership is often lauded but at times, difficult to put into everyday practice. How can we treat each staff member as a unique individual who deserves our total respect and attention? How can a nurse manager be a risk taker who uses creativity to approach complex problems? What kind of vision must you articulate to engage and motivate your employees? Inspiring others to trust and follow you takes a special type of communication and cognition, and acting as a worthy role model even when you might like to kick back and to be in the passenger seat for a while can be exhausting.

There is much to be said for the collective wisdom of nurses. Receiving advice and feedback from a group of "expert" managers, much as you might consult with a colleague over coffee or away from work, is a unique opportunity. While you might not see the scenarios described as particularly problematic or agree with the advice or solutions the respondents offered, it's helpful to have a "real life" perspective on conflict in the workplace. Both nurse managers and individual staff who struggle to understand the rationale of those in positions of oversight can use the reflections, summaries, activities, and appendices to learn more about themselves and those they work with.

This is how our profession develops and improves. When nurses help nurses, we will not only survive but thrive in a time of both crisis and opportunity.

part VI appendixes

A | is your management style causing conflict?

Circle the statements below that you feel describe you as a manager.

1. If there's a minor interpersonal problem among staff, I don't get involved.

2. When a particular staff member irritates me, I try to avoid him/her as much as possible without jeopardizing patient care.

3. One of the things that bothers me the most at work is having to "pick up after" team members who don't do their jobs the way they should.

4. I go out of my way to spontaneously check in with staff throughout the day and make an effort to follow up on any issues.

5. Some staff members require an authoritarian management style so I treat them accordingly.

6. If I'm upset with a coworker, I'm more likely to email him or her about it than speak face to face.

7. When there's an issue about some aspect of patient care, I usually take the suggestions of the nurses who have been there the longest.

8. During conversations with staff, I sometimes share a little bit of information about my home life.

9. The nurse who works the hardest gets the biggest pay increase from me.

10. There have been times when I raised my voice or spoke harshly to make a point to my staff.

If you haven't already figured out the desired answers, 1, 4, and 8 would be behaviors that most likely *wouldn't* cause conflict. Statements 2, 3, 5, 6, 7, 9, and 10 most likely *would* cause conflict. For all the statements, the ones you *agreed* with are a place to begin adjusting your management style. An especially mature nurse manager can expect that staff or supervisors who rate him or her with this tool will match self-rated responses pretty closely.

B | conflict case scenario

Maya is the nurse manager of a busy medical step-down unit in a suburban community hospital. She obtained her BSN 2 years ago after working for 5 years as an LPN on the same floor she now manages.

Seleena, a young AD nurse who has recently relocated to the area for the school system, has only worked on the unit for 8 months. She tends to keep to herself and spend her downtime talking to her children on her personal phone. Sometimes the other nurses have a hard time getting Seleena to answer her patients' call bells in a timely manner, which has gotten steadily more noticeable. The CNAs also complain that Seleena is condescending and bossy.

One afternoon Laurena, Maya's supervisor, pulls her aside. "You have a problem," she says. "We've gotten some anonymous complaints about Seleena. They came right to the CEO, and he told me to 'take care of it.' What's going on?"

Maya is defensive. "What did the complaints say?"

"That she's lazy and doesn't pull her weight. They were clearly from coworkers. There've been some patient satisfaction surveys for your unit that weren't too good, either."

"OK, I'll take care of it," Maya says.

With a sinking heart, Maya summons Seleena into her office at the end of the workday and tells her, "We need to talk. There have been some complaints about things here on the floor."

"Don't you get it?" Seleena says, shaking her head.

"What? Do you know something I don't?" Maya asks.

"You and I are the only people of color here. The nurses here treat both of us like dirt, and it doesn't take a lot of brainpower to figure out why. They think they're better than us."

Maya doesn't know how to respond. As she thinks about it, she has to agree that the nurses on the floor seem to act a little more respectful to Laurena than they do to her.

What are the key problems Maya needs to address?

Did Laurena handle the feedback she received correctly?

How should Seleena's comments be treated?

Is there a need for a unit-wide intervention, and if so, what would it be?

C | organizational cynicism self-assessment

The following questions are adapted from an organizational cynicism scale developed by James Wilkerson and his colleagues for use in research studies (Wilkerson, Evans, & Davis, 2008). We've modified it here to provide an informal way to gauge your "OC quotient."

If you read the statements and find yourself nodding your head and strongly agreeing with the sentiments, then you are probably organizationally cynical. The more questions you agree with—and the strength of your agreement—will tell you just *how* organizationally cynical you are.

1. Efforts to make things better at my organization are unlikely to succeed.

2. The management at my company is not very good at running improvement programs or making other necessary changes.

3. Overall, I expect more disappointments than successes in working with this company.

4. My company doesn't pull its fair share of the weight in its relationship with its employees.

5. Suggestions about how to solve problems around here don't usually promote much real change.

6. I don't feel that my company meets my expectations for quality of work life.

7. Company management is more interested in its goals and needs than its employees' welfare.

8. My employer does not care about me as an individual or support my efforts to succeed.

9. The organization where I work really doesn't care much about patients or employees.

10. There aren't many times when I feel proud of working in my current job.

D | when it's time to seek outside counsel

–J. Stephen Woodside, Esquire

The relational conflicts and bullying described in this important book raise serious concerns about the workplace. Productivity drops, absenteeism and turnover increase, departments and entire organizations suffer, and management falls short of goals and objectives, laying the groundwork for more tension and blame. Quite often, the employee may consider to filing a lawsuit or an employment charge. The desire to sue becomes a consuming process, feeding into the cycle of tension instead of rectifying it.

How can the targeted employee or manager know when he or she may have a lawsuit or claim? While the elements of a legal claim in the employment setting are complicated and beyond the scope of this discussion, the types of conflicts and issues raised in this book may have a connection to such a claim, and in some cases (depending on the severity of the conduct and required elements in the residing state), a legal claim might arise out of the conduct alone.

In the employment setting, adverse action, bad acts or words, and aggressive or degrading conduct between employees and their supervisors often masks or is part of an underlying intention or desire to harass, inflict distress, or discriminate against the employee—an unlawful means to achieve an unlawful end. While a bright line may not be drawn between relational bullying behavior and a legal claim, there are specific actions that may indicate discrimination, unlawful harassment, or infliction of emotional distress is afoot *and* a legal claim might exist. In these situations, the employee (or manager) may want to consult with an attorney.

The following checklist presents some of the more common indicators both the employee and employer should be aware of that might connect a relationally aggressive or hostile employer or employee (or workplace) to possible actionable conduct and a legal claim. The list is not exhaustive. The list is not legal opinion or advice but should serve as a reference guide to assist the reader within the specific context of the material presented. The items are in no particular order of importance or weight. Always, the reader should consult with an attorney of his or her choice who is knowledgeable of the applicable laws within the residing state.

Checklist

1. Wages or salary are reduced.

2. Wage or salary increases are denied.

3. Work shift is changed or adjusted, leading to reduced wages or salary.

4. Wages, salary, or benefits due and owing are unpaid.

5. Benefits (defined in the broadest sense) are decreased or materially changed.

6. Benefits (defined in the broadest sense) are eliminated or denied.

7. Overtime hours or shift hours are reduced, leading to reduced wages or salary.

8. Overtime shift/schedule is changed, eliminated, or interrupted, leading to reduced overtime hours/pay.

9. Work shift is changed, eliminated, or interrupted, leading to reduced hours/pay.

10. Employee is moved, transferred, or rotated out of the unit, floor, or department; pay or benefits are reduced.

11. Job, position, rank, or title is eliminated.

12. Job duties within position, rank, or title are materially reduced, changed, or eliminated.

13. Working conditions within a particular job classification or title are materially changed or worsened.

14. Employee is transferred to another position, unit, or floor to perform duties of employees junior or less tenured.

15. Employee is demoted in position by organizational structure, title, or name.

16. Scheduled promotion is denied, materially delayed, or altered in content or duration.

17. Employment is terminated.

18. Employee is cajoled or pushed into retirement or "early retirement."

19. Repeated requests or applications for promotion, reassignment, transfer, pay or benefits increases, reimbursements, shift changes, etc., are refused, ignored, or "lost."

20. Job training or education is refused or blocked, threatening or preventing advancement.

21. Job skill, policy, or compliance updates or materials are refused or blocked, threatening or hindering work performance or career advancement.

22. Employee is required or urged to come in early, stay late, skip breaks, skip lunch, or work on days off without full or partial compensation for all or any of this time.

23. A medical condition, disability, or mental or physical condition or impairment is ignored, not accommodated, or not considered or addressed by the employer.

24. Performance reviews or evaluations are refused, scheduled late, ignored, or noncompliant in some material way.

25. Performance reviews or evaluations contain false or misleading data or information or are altered or amended in some material way.

26. Print, writings, pictures, or signs are used in the workplace to ridicule, mock, scorn, or degrade the employee or to incite hatred or opinion against the employee.

27. Oral statements, expressions, or transitory gestures are used to ridicule, mock, scorn, or degrade the employee or to incite hatred or opinion against the employee.

28. Employee is the target of unwanted physical or sexual contact or advances.

29. Employee is the target of sexual innuendo, comments, jokes, writings, words, pictures, or other sexual materials.

30. Employee is subjected in the work environment to sexual innuendo, comments, jokes, writings, words, pictures, or other sexual materials.

31. Employee reports the type of material, content, or environment under nos. 26–30 above to supervisory personnel, and no responsive action is taken.

32. Employee is subject to an abusive, hostile, or harassing gender-driven work environment (not necessarily sexual), and the conduct is severe and regular.

33. Employee is the subject or target of a *quid pro quo* arrangement—sex in exchange for favorable work or conditions, position, pay, benefits, or promotion, etc.

34. Employee is asked or told to perform or participate in any act or omission that could constitute a HIPAA violation.

35. Employee is asked or told to perform or participate in any act or omission that could constitute a violation of the employer's stated policies, procedures, or protocols.

36. Employee is the target or subject, directly or indirectly, of stray comments or words, gossip, or innuendo that raise age, race, gender, sex, religious, national origin, medical, or disability considerations, *and* one or more of the types of adverse employment actions above might also be present.

37. Access to the bargaining unit (union) stewards or representatives, or to the bargaining unit process, is delayed, hindered, or denied in some material way.

As noted earlier, the reader should consult with an attorney of his or her choice who is knowledgeable of the applicable laws within the residing state.

J. Stephan Woodside is an attorney experienced in employment litigation. His practice is based in the Philadelphia, Pennsylvania, area. He can be reached at jstephanwood@verizon.net

references

Allen, N. J., & Meyer, J. P. (1996). Affective, continuance, and normative commitment to the organization: An examination of construct validity. *Journal of Vocational Behavior, 49*(3), 252–276.

Almost, J., Doran, D., McGillis Hall, L., & Spence Laschinger, H. (2010). Antecedents and consequences of intragroup conflict among nurses. *Journal of Nursing Management, 18,* 981–992.

American Association of Colleges of Nursing (AACN). (2012). *Violence as a public health problem.* Position statement: Workplace violence prevention. Washington, DC: Author.

American Nurses Association (ANA). (2012). Bullying and workplace violence. *NursingWorld.* Silver Spring, MD: Author.

Andrews, M. E., Stewart, N. J., Morgan, D. G., & D'Arcy, C. (2012). More alike than different: A comparison of male and female RNs in rural and remote Canada. *Journal of Nursing Management, 20*(4), 561–570.

Armour, S. (2005). Do women compete in unhealthy ways at work? *USA Today.* Retrieved from http://www.usatoday.com/money/workplace/2005-12-29-women-bosses-usat_x.htm

Barrett, A., Korber, S., Padula, C., & Piatek, C. (2009, October/December). Lessons learned from a lateral violence and team building intervention. *Nursing Administration Quarterly, 33*(4), 342–351.

Barton, S., Alamri, M., Cella, D., Cherry, K., Curil, K., Hallman, B., ... & Zuraikat, N. (2011, August). Dissolving clique behavior. *Nursing Management, 42*(8), 32–37.

Bedeian, A. G. (2007). Even if the tower is "ivory," it isn't "white": Understanding the consequences of faculty cynicism. *Academy of Management Learning & Education, 6*(1), 9–32.

Beilock, S. (2011, August). Word of mouth: What makes us gossip? *Psychology Today.* Retrieved from http://www.psychologytoday.com/blog/choke/201108/word-mouth-what-makes-us-gossip

Berger, J. (2011). Arousal increases social transmission of information. *Psychological Science, 22*(7), 891–893.

Casserly, M. (2012). When snitches get stitches: Physical violence as workplace retaliation on the rise. *Forbes Magazine.* Retrieved from http://www.forbes.com/sites/meghancasserly/2012/09/21/when-snitches-get-stitches-physical-violence-as-workplace-retaliation-on-the-rise/

Catalyst. (2012, September). *High potentials in the pipeline: Leaders pay it forward.* [Powerpoint slides].

Cell phones: On-duty Facebook posting violated rules, nurse's firing upheld. (2011, June). *Legal Eagle Eye Newsletter.* Retrieved from http://www.nursinglaw.com/facebook.pdf

Ceravolo, D. J., Schwartz, D. G., Foltz-Ramos, K. M., & Castner, J. (2012). Strengthening communication to overcome lateral violence. *Journal of Nursing Management, 20*(5), 599–606.

Dean, J. W., Brandes, P., & Dharwadkar, R. (1998). Organizational cynicism. *The Academy of Management Review, 23*(2), 341–352.

Dehue, F., Bolman, C., Vollink, T., & Mouwelse, M. (2012). Coping with bullying at work and health related problems. *International Journal of Stress Management, 19*(3), 175–197.

Dellasega, C. (2009). Bullying among nurses. *American Journal of Nursing, 112*(9), 52–58.

Dellasega, C. (2011). *When nurses hurt nurses: Recognizing and overcoming the cycle of nurse bullying.* Indianapolis, IN: Sigma Theta Tau International.

Dellasega, C., Gabbay, R., Durdock, K., & Martinez-King, N. (2009). An exploratory study of the orientation needs of experienced nurses. *The Journal of Continuing Education in Nursing, 40*(7), 311–316.

DeMaria, J. (2011, July 4). 3 male nurse myths. *Scrubs: The Nurse's Guide to Good Living.* Retrieved from http://scrubsmag.com/male-nurse-myths/

Diller, V. (2012, April). Female competition as we age: Who's the fairest one of all? *Psychology Today.* Retrieved from http://www.psychologytoday.com/blog/face-it/201204/female-competition-we-age-whos-the-fairest-one-all

Ellingston, L. (2002). Communication, collaboration, and teamwork among health care professionals. *Communication Research Trends, 21*(3), 2–17.

Evans, J. (1997). Men in nursing: Issues of gender segregation and hidden advantage. [Review]. *Journal of Advanced Nursing, 26*(2), 226–231.

Felblinger, D. M. (2008). Incivility and bullying in the workplace and nurses' shame responses. [Review]. *Journal of Obstetric, Gynecologic, and Neonatal Nursing, 37*(2), 234-241; quiz 241–242.

Fuller, R. (2010, July). Somebodies and nobodies: 10 ways to stop rankism in the professional world. *Psychology Today*. Retrieved from http://www.psychologytoday.com/blog/somebodies-and-nobodies/201002/what-is-rankism-and-why-do-we-do-it

Gaffney, D., Demarco, R., Hofmeyer, A., Vessey, J., & Budin, W. (2012). Making things right: Nurses' experience with workplace bullying—a grounded theory. *Nursing Research & Practice*, *2012*, article ID 243210.

Gardner, D. (2005, January). Ten lessons in collaboration. *OJIN: The Online Journal of Issues in Nursing*, *10*(1), Manuscript 1.

Gessler, R., & Ferron, L. (2012, April). When caregiving ignites burnout—New ways to douse the flames. *American Nurse Today*, *7*(4). Retrieved from http://www.americannursetoday/article.aspx?id=8980&fid=8916

Gray, E. (2012, May 6). Women at work: Jealousy and envy impact women differently than men. *Huffington Post*. Retrieved from http://www.huffingtonpost.com/emma-gray/women-at-work-jealousy-envy-men_b_1480030.html

Grosser, T., Lopez-Kidwell, V., & Labianca, G. (2010). A social network analysis of positive and negative gossip in organizational life. *Group & Organization Management*, *35*, 1–36.

Hader, R. (2010). Nurse leaders: A closer look. *Nursing Management*, *41*(1), 25–29. doi: 10.1097/01.NUMA.0000366900.80524.d4

How to handle office politics. (2012). *The Wall Street Journal*. Retrieved from http://guides.wsj.com/careers/how-to-overcome-career-obstacles/how-to-handle-office-politics/

Hrobsky, P., & Kersbergen, A. (2002, December). Preceptors' perceptions of clinical performance failure. *Journal of Nursing Education*, *41*(12), 550–553.

Hutchinson, M., Jackson, D., Wilkes, L., & Vickers, M. (2008). A new model of bullying in the nursing workplace. *Advances in Nursing Science, 31*(2), 860–[871.

Institute of Medicine. (1999). *To err is human: Building a safer health system.* Washington, DC: Author.

Institute of Medicine. (2001). *Crossing the quality chasm: A new health system for the 21st century* [Consensus report]. Washington, DC: National Academies Press.

Institute of Medicine. (2005). *Keeping patients safe: Transforming the work environment of nurses.* Washington, DC: National Academies Press.

Johansen, M. (2012, February). Keeping the peace: Conflict management strategies for nurse managers. *Nursing Management, 43*(2), 50–54.

Kalish, B., Lee, H., & Rochman, M. (2010). Nursing staff teamwork and job satisfaction. *Journal of Nursing Management, 18*, 938–947.

Kauffman, G. (2012). *Teaching millennials.* Presentation on *Distinguished Educators of Penn State College of Medicine.* The Milton S. Hershey Medical Center/Pennsylvania State College of Medicine.

Kearns, S. (2010, February 9). Half of nurses plan career change, says survey. *HealthLeaders Media.* Retrieved from http://www.healthleadersmedia.com/page-1/NRS-246272/Half-of-Nurses-Plan-Career-Change-Says-Survey

Kim, T. Y., Bateman, T. S., Gilbreth, B., & Anderson, L. M. (2009). Top management credibility and employee cynicism: A comprehensive model. *Human Relations, 62*, 1435–1458.

Lally, R. (2009). Bullies aren't only on the playground: A look at nurse-on-nurse violence. *ONS Connect, 24*(2), 17.

Lee, H., Spiers, J., Yurtseven, O., Cummings, G., Sharlow, J. Bhatti, S., & Germann, P. (2010). Impact of leadership development on emotional health in healthcare managers. *Journal of Nursing Management, 18,* 1027–1039.

Luczwek, D. R. (2007). Can personality buffer cynicism? Moderating effects of extraversion and neuroticism in response to workplace hassles. *Dissertation Abstracts International: Section B: The Sciences and Engineering, 68*(2-B), 1350.

Marlantes, L. (2011, January 13). After the Arizona shooting, the civility movement sees tipping point. *The Christian Science Monitor.*

Maryland State Board of Nursing (MSBN). (2005, August). *Civility in the workplace.* Baltimore, MD: Maryland Nursing Workforce Commission 21215-2254. Retrieved from http://www.mbon.org/commission/workplace_ civility.ppt

McCloughen, A., O'Brien, L., & Jackson, D. (2009). Esteemed connection: Creating a mentoring relationship for nurse leadership. *Nursing Inquiry, 16*(4), 326–336.

Mooney, N. (2005). *I can't believe she did that!: Why women betray other women at work.* New York, NY: Saint Martin's Press.

National Advisory Council on Nurse Education and Practice (NACNEP). (2007, December). *Violence against nurses: An assessment of the causes and impacts of violence in nursing education and practice.* Fifth annual report to the Secretary of the U.S. Department of Health and Human Services and the U.S. Congress. Washington, DC: Author.

National Council of State Boards of Nursing (NCSBN). (2011, August). A nurse's guide to the use of social media. Chicago, IL: Author. Retrieved from https:// www.ncsbn.org/3487.htm

Naus, F., van Iterson, A., & Roe, R. (2007). Organizational cynicism: Extending the exit, voice, loyalty and neglect model of employees' responses to adverse conditions in the workplace. *Human Relations, 60*, 683–718.

Okey Eneh, V., Vehvilainen-Julkunen, K., & Kvist, T. (2012). Nursing leadership practices as perceived by Finnish nursing staff: High ethics, less feedback and rewards. *Journal of Nursing Management, 20*, 159–169.

Orloff, J. (2005). *Positive energy: 10 extraordinary prescriptions for transforming fatigue, stress, and fear into vibrance, strength, and love.* New York, NY: Three Rivers Press.

Regan, L., & Rodriguez, L. (2011, Winter). Nurse empowerment from a middle-management perspective: Nurse managers' and assistant nurse managers' workplace empowerment views. *The Permanente Journal, 15*(1).

Rousseau, D., & Tijoriwala, S. (1999). What's a good reason to change? Motivated reasoning and social accounts in promoting organizational change. *Journal of Applied Psychology, 84*(4), 514–528.

Rubin, R. S., Dierdorff, E. C., Bommer, W. H., & Baldwin, T. T. (2009). Do leaders reap what they sow? Leader and employee outcomes of leader organizational cynicism about change. *The Leadership Quarterly, 20*(5), 680–688.

Rushton, C. H., Reina, M. L., Francovich, C., Naumann, P., & Reina, D. S. (2010). Application of the Reina Trust and Betrayal Model to the experience of pediatric critical care clinicians. *American Journal of Critical Care, 19*(4), e41–51.

Russell, J. (2012, June). Cultivating civility in the workplace. *The Washington Post.* Retrieved from http://www.washingtonpost.com/business/capitalbusiness/career-coach-how-to-cultivate-civility-in-the-workplace/2012/06/15/gJQA6YIjjV_story.html

Schalk, R. (2011). The influence of organizational commitment and health on sickness absenteeism: A longitudinal study. *Journal of Nursing Management, 19*(5), 596–600.

Schwehm, K. (2006, July). *Civility in the workplace*. [Powerpoint slides]. Louisiana State University. Retrieved from http://www.docstoc.com/docs/109810918/CivilityintheWorkplace

Shapiro Barash, S. (2006). *Tripping the prom queen*. New York, NY: St. Martin's Press.

Simons, S. (2008). Workplace bullying experienced by Massachusetts registered nurses and the relationship to intention to leave the organization. *Advances in Nursing Science, 31*(2), E48–E59.

Smith, M. (2011, September). Magnet hospital: Are you a transformational leader? *Nursing Management, 42*(9), 44–50.

Sparks, A. M. (2012). Psychological empowerment and job satisfaction between Baby Boomer and Generation X nurses. *Journal of Nursing Management, 20*(4), 451–460.

Spence Laschinger, H. K. (2010). Positive working relationships matter for better nurse and patient outcomes. *Journal of Nursing Management, 18*, 875–877.

Spence Laschinger, H. K., & Leiter, M. P. (2006). The impact of nursing work environments on patient safety outcomes: The mediating role of burnout/engagement. *The Journal of Nursing Administration, 36*(5), 259–267.

Tema, T. R., Poggenpoel, M., & Myburgh, C. P. (2011). Experiences of psychiatric nurses exposed to hostility from patients in a forensic ward. *Journal of Nursing Management, 19*(7), 915–924.

Townsend, T. (2012, January). Break the bullying cycle. *American Nurse Today, 7*(1). Retrieved from http://www.americannursetoday.com/article.aspx?id=8648&fid=8612

U.S. Department of Health and Human Services, HRSA. (2010). *The registered nurse population; Initial findings from the 2008 National Sample Survey of Registered Nurses.*

U.S. Department of Labor, Bureau of Labor Statistics. (2012, September). Occupational outlook handbook, 2012-13: Registered nurses. Retrieved from http://www.bls.gov/ooh/healthcare/registered-nurses.htm

Valentine, P. (1995, July). Management of conflict: Do nurses/women handle it differently? *Journal of Advanced Nursing, 22*(1), 142–149.

Vessey, J., DeMarco, R., Gaffney, D., & Budin, W. (2009, September/October). Bullying of staff registered nurses in the workplace: A preliminary study for developing personal and organizational strategies for the transformation of hostile to healthy workplace environments. *Journal of Professional Nursing, 25*(5), 299–306.

The WBI definition of workplace bullying. (2012). *The Workplace Bullying Institute.* Retrieved from http://www.workplacebullying.org/individuals/problem/definition/

Wilkerson, J. M., Evans, W. R., & Davis, W. D. (2008). A test of coworkers' influence on organizational cynicism, badmouthing, and organizational citizenship behavior. *Journal of Applied Social Psychology, 38*(9), 2273–2292.

Wilson, A. (2005, April/June). Impact of management development on nurse retention. *Nursing Administration Quarterly, 29*(2), 137–145.

Yamada, D. (2008, Summer). Workplace bullying and ethical leadership. *The Journal of JVBL: Values-Based Leadership, 1*(2), 49–62.

Yildirim, D. (2009). Bullying among nurses and its effects. *International Nursing Review, 56*, 504–511.

Younge, O., Hagler, P., Cox, C., & Drefs, S. (2008, May/ June). Time to truly acknowledge what nursing preceptors do for students. *Journal for Nurses in Staff Development, 24*(3), 113–116.

Zastocki, D., & Holly, C. (2010, December). Retaining nurse managers. *American Nurse Today, 5*(12).

index of vignettes

index of commentators

index

Colleague Recognition Day,
189–190

commentators. *See* Index of
Commentators, page 323

commitment to nursing
position, 274–275

communication. *See also*
gossip
about institutional change,
38, 40, 199–201, 268
about mergers, 197–198
and chain of command,
216, 285
closed-loop
communication, 178
collaboration and, 178
competition and, 93
conflict and lack of
communication, 163
constructive *versus*
destructive
communication, 284–
285
during crisis situations,
186–187
criticism and, 25–27
cyberbullying, 48–50
empowering
communication, 283
facilitated meetings, 143
misdirected
communication, 95
negative talk, 276–278
negative *versus* positive,
212–214
with patients, 235–236
professional *versus*
unprofessional, 51–52
relationships and, 141,
209

sharing intimate details, 93
in shift reports, 151–154
technology and, 51–53
and top-down changes,
199–201, 268

competition
beneficial aspects of, 100
between colleagues, 152
communication and, 93
versus cooperation, 157
friendly competition,
103–104
getting along, 92
rivalry among units, 139
in salary and promotions,
91–92, 99–100
scarcity of executive
positions, 93
in upward mobility, 92
between women, 92,
140–141

complaints
about nursing care, 233–
236
complaint box, 241
legitimate complaints
versus "artifacts of
resentment," 236
staff, 30

confidentiality, 46–47
managers and, 127
versus privacy, 106

conflict journal, 222

conflict-management
techniques
confidence in, 240
enhancing collaboration,
176
identifying bullying,
25–27